. . the
juices &
smoothies
bible

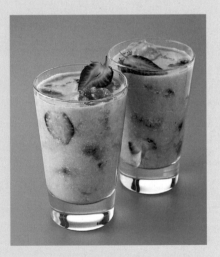

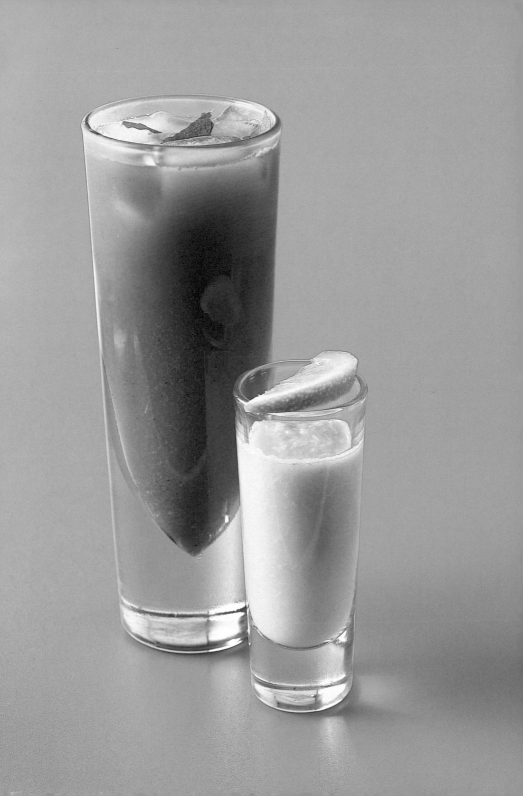

. . the
juices &
smoothies
bible

over 150 recipes for a healthy lifestyle

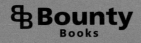

Bounty
Books

First published in 2014 by Bounty Books, a division of Octopus Publishing Group Ltd

Reprinted in 2015 by Bounty Books, a division of Octopus Publishing Group Ltd, Carmelite House, 50 Victoria Embankment London EC4Y 0DZ www.octopusbooks.co.uk

An Hachette UK Company www.hachette.co.uk

ISBN 978-0-753727-31-7

Printed and bound in China

Publisher: Samantha Warrington
Editorial and Design Manager: Emma Hill
Editor: Jane Birch
Designer: Chris Bell/cbdesign
Production Manager: Pete Hunt

contents

introduction

Juices and smoothies provide the delicious, easy and fast way to consume a wide range of good-for-you fruit and vegetables for all-round health and vitality.

getting the most from this book

This comprehensive collection of over 150 flavour-packed juices and smoothies is divided into three handy sections so – whether you want to boost energy levels, detoxify your system or simply quench your thirst – you can choose the recipe that suits your needs.

- **daily** (see page 12) contains smoothies for meals on the run, juices to tempt reluctant veg-eaters and other mouthwatering blends of fruit and veg to enjoy every day, all year round.
- **healthy** (see page 72) are recipes that target specific ailments, such as asthma and high blood pressure, and provide the vitamins and minerals you need at certain times, including during pregnancy or when dieting.
- **energy** juices and smoothies (see page 132) are ideal for sports people, giving an extra boost before, during and after exercise.

Before you turn to the recipes, here are some juicing basics to get you started.

why make your own juices?

Fresh, home-made juices surpass anything you can buy from supermarkets or even health food stores. Bought juices usually contain additives and preservatives and many don't have much fresh juice in them at all. By making your own, you can choose exactly what ingredients to use, and you have the peace of mind of knowing exactly where they came from.

For maximum benefit, drink juices immediately after you've made them as the ingredients deteriorate fast once juiced. If you don't, store leftovers in the refrigerator and consume within 24 hours.

choosing and preparing ingredients

The quality of a juice is directly related to the freshness of the ingredients. Try to use the best you can get, always choosing those with good colour and optimum ripeness. Organic produce is free from chemical residues and, although it's more expensive, devotees swear by the improved taste and juiciness.

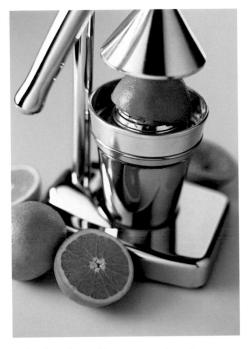

Organic ingredients need not be peeled, which is desirable as most vitamins and minerals tend to be lie just below the surface of fruit and vegetable skins (which is also where pesticide residues collect). Prepare ingredients just before using them so that fewer nutrients are lost through oxidization.

Although fresh is usually best, if fruit and vegetables are frozen soon after picking they can be better than fresh produce that is past its best. Summer fruits – strawberries, blueberries and raspberries – are a good example. If you use canned fruit, make sure it is in natural juice or water, not syrup. Dried fruits, in particular apricots, prunes and dates, are a concentrated source of sugars, vitamins and minerals but soak them overnight to make them easier to purée.

to peel or not to peel

Most enzymes, vitamins and minerals lie just below the skins of fruits and vegetables, so include them where possible. If you use organic produce you can leave most skins on, but remember to wash each item thoroughly in warm water first. Generally, it is safer to peel non-organic produce. Always

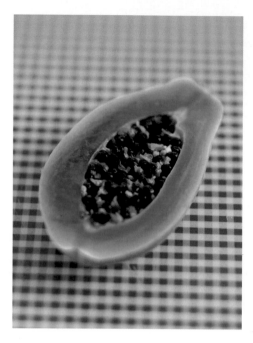

peel avocados, bananas, mangoes, papaya and pineapple. You can leave the skin on unwaxed citrus fruits if some rind is called for in the recipe, but it is more usual to peel them, or squeeze them in a lemon squeezer. Leave the skin on kiwifruit unless the recipe states otherwise.

remove stones and seeds

Remove large stones such as those in apricots, avocados, mangoes, peaches and plums. Many melon seeds are full of juice, so unless instructed otherwise, include them, with the exception of papaya seeds. Apple and citrus seeds may make the juice bitter, so don't put them in.

other ingredients

Other ingredients such as milk, yogurt, nuts, seeds and herbal teas make for even more interesting and nutritious drinks. Some recipes contain supplements, which are a concentrated source of essential vitamins and minerals. Spirulina is a form of chlorophyll credited with, among other benefits, halting the signs of ageing. It is good in juices but may spoil their colour. Energizing wheatgrass is also rich in chlorophyll and boosts immunity.

be creative

Once you have tried some of these recipes, do not be afraid to experiment with some of your own, but follow these simple guidelines:

- carrots and apples blend well with almost anything.
- avoid too many strong-tasting vegetables in one juice.
- if using strong- or bitter-tasting vegetables, dilute and sweeten them with carrot and cucumber.

juicing equipment

You may already own a lemon squeezer and a food processor or blender, but to make the juices in this book you will also need to invest in a specialist juicer which can separate the juice from the pulp of most fruits and vegetables. When choosing, select one that has a big enough opening for larger fruit and vegetables, and one that comes apart for easy cleaning.

types of juicer

- **citrus juicer:** commonly known as the humble lemon squeezer, it's ideal for extracting the juice from lemons, limes, oranges and grapefruit. Citrus fruits can be peeled (leaving as much pith on as possible) and juiced as other ingredients if you prefer. Citrus juices are highly acidic and are best diluted, either with other juices or water.
- **centrifugal juicer:** the most widely available and affordable of the specialized juicers on the market: ingredients are fed into a rapidly spinning grater which separates the pulp from the juice by centrifugal force.
- **masticating juicer:** this type is more expensive but gives a higher yield. The ingredients are pulverized and forced through a fine wire mesh to extract the maximum amount of liquid.
- **food processor or blender:** this works by puréeing ingredients and is used to make smoothies, as well as to mix crushed ice into some juices. Make sure your blender or food processor is strong enough to crush ice; if it is not, you can use ice-cold water instead.

cleaning your juicer

Clean your juicer thoroughly each time it is used to prevent bacterial growth on any pulp residues. Look for a machine that dismantles easily so that cleaning does not become an annoying task. Soak the equipment in warm soapy water and use a new toothbrush or nail brush to get into any awkward corners. A solution of one part white vinegar to two parts water will reduce staining and discoloration.

Juices and smoothies should be used a part of a sensible eating plan so you should still eat enough from the other food groups (including grains, dairy foods and protein). If you are following a special diet or are under medical supervision, consult your health practitioner before making drastic changes to your health regime.

great ingredients

apple rich in: beta-carotene, folic acid, vitamin C, calcium, magnesium, phosphorus, potassium, pectin. **also:** copper, zinc and vitamins B1, B2, B3, B6 and E.

apricot rich in: beta-carotene, vitamin C, papain, calcium, magnesium, phosphorus, potassium, flavonoids. **also:** B vitamins, iron, zinc.

artichoke (globe) rich in: magnesium, phosphorus, potassium, sodium, folic acid, beta-carotene, vitamin B3, vitamin C, vitamin K.

avocado rich in: vitamin E, potassium, monounsaturated fat, vitamin B.

banana rich in: beta-carotene, vitamin C, folic acid, magnesium, calcium, phosphorus, potassium. **also:** iron, B vitamins, zinc.

beetroot rich in: folate, folic acid, soluble fibre.

blackberry rich in: beta-carotene, vitamins C and E, calcium, magnesium, phosphorus, potassium, sodium.

blackcurrant rich in: beta-carotene, vitamins C and E, calcium, magnesium, phosphorus, potassium. **also:** B vitamins, copper, iron.

broccoli rich in: beta-carotene, folate, vitamin C, potassium, iron.

brussels sprouts rich in: potassium, beta-carotene, folate, vitamin C.

cabbage rich in: vitamin C, folate, beta-carotene and fibre.

carrot rich in: beta-carotene and alpha-carotene.

celery rich in: phytonutrients and apiin.

cherry rich in: beta-carotene, vitamin C, folic acid, calcium, magnesium, phosphorus, potassium, flavonoids.

chives rich in: plant chemicals.

cinnamon we don't eat a large enough amounts of spices to receive nutrients from them.

coriander (ground) we don't eat a large enough quantity of spices to receive nutrients from them.

cranberry rich in: vitamin C, potassium, carotene, fibre.

cucumber rich in: potassium, beta-carotene, silicon, sulphur, sodium, phosphorus.

dandelion rich in: iron, copper.

endive rich in: potassium, beta-carotene, folate.

fennel rich in: vitamin C.

garlic rich in: potassium, calcium, magnesium.

ginger rich in: zinc, selenium.

grape rich in: glucose, fructose, potassium, vitamin C, carotene.

grapefruit rich in: vitamin C, potassium, calcium, carotenes, folate.

horseradish rich in: potassium, calcium, folate, vitamin C.

jerusalem artichoke rich in: potassium, niacin, inutase, inulin.

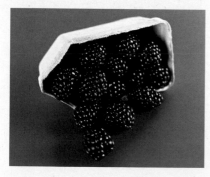

kale rich in: beta-carotene, folate, calcium, potassium.

lemon rich in: vitamin C, potassium, calcium, fructose.

lettuce rich in: beta-carotene, folate, potassium.

lime rich in: vitamin C, potassium, carotenes and calcium.

live natural yogurt rich in: calcium, vitamin D.

mango rich in: vitamin C, carotenes, fibre and B vitamins.

melon rich in: calcium, magnesium, potassium, phosphorus, vitamin C, beta-carotene.

milk rich in: protein, zinc, phosphorus, B vitamins and vitamin A. Soya milk is an alternative to cows' milk but, as it naturally lacks calcium, it is better to choose a brand fortified with calcium

mint rich in: calcium, iron, magnesium, folate.

onion rich in: antioxidants, potassium, calcium.

orange rich in: vitamin C, potassium, carotene, lutein.

papaya rich in: vitamin C, antioxidants, potassium.

parsley rich in: vitamin C.

parsnip rich in: niacin, B vitamins, folate and vitamin C.

peach rich in: antioxidant carotenes, flavonoids and vitamin C.

peanut butter rich in: protein, fibre, vitamin E, B vitamins, copper and magnesium. **also:** contains phytochemicals.

pear rich in: potassium, beta-carotene, vitamin C.

pineapple rich in: antioxidant vitamin C, bromelain, potassium, beta-carotene.

potato rich in: potassium, fibre, folate, vitamin C, carotenes and calcium.

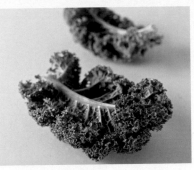

prunes rich in: fibre, potassium, iron, calcium, beta-carotene.

radish rich in: calcium, potassium, folate.

raspberry rich in: phytonutrient ellagic acid, magnesium, potassium, vitamin C.

soya rich in: calcium and protein.

spinach rich in: iron, folate, beta-carotene, calcium.

strawberry rich in: vitamin C, potassium, calcium, magnesium, phosphorus.

sweet potato rich in: vitamin C, vitamin E, beta-carotene.

tomato rich in: vitamin C, fibre, lycopene, beta-carotene, potassium, folate.

turnip rich in: iron, beta-carotene, vitamin B, vitamin C.

watercress rich in: iron, vitamin C, beta-carotene.

watermelon rich in: beta-carotene, folic acid, vitamin B5, vitamin C, calcium, magnesium, phosphorus, potassium.

yam rich in: potassium, calcium, folate, fibre.

yogurt rich in: calcium, potassium, protein and vitamin B12. **also:** many contain probiotics for a healthy digestive system.

daily

Fruit and vegetables contain many of the important enzymes, vitamins and minerals that we need to stay healthy and full of vitality. Juicing several types of raw fruit and vegetables daily is a simple and super-tasty way to ensure you receive your full quota of these vital nutrients. This chapter has recipes for meal-in-a-glass smoothies, refreshing fruit blends and mouthwatering concoctions to make even vegetable-loathing toddlers happy.

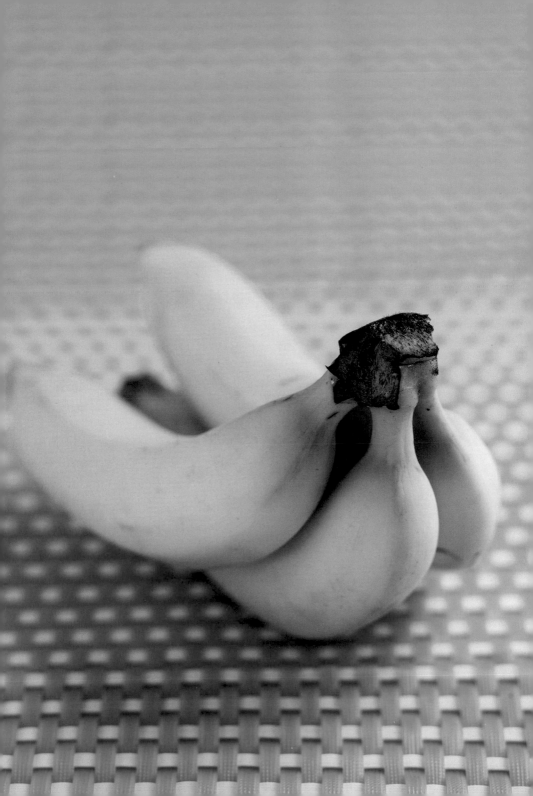

beetroot, grape & orange

2 small beetroot, about 100g (3½ oz)
50 g (2 oz) grapes
1 orange

Juice all ingredients and serve in a tumbler with ice to chill. Decorate with an orange slice, if liked.

makes 200 ml (7 fl oz)

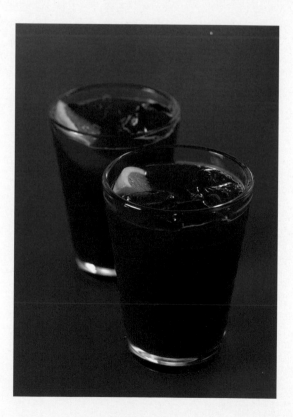

breakfast smoothie

250 ml (8 fl oz) semi-skimmed milk
½ large banana
½ large mango
1 tablespoon peanut butter

Blend together all the ingredients with a couple of ice cubes for a silky,
satisfying smoothie. To serve decorate with slices of mango.

makes 300 ml (10 fl oz)

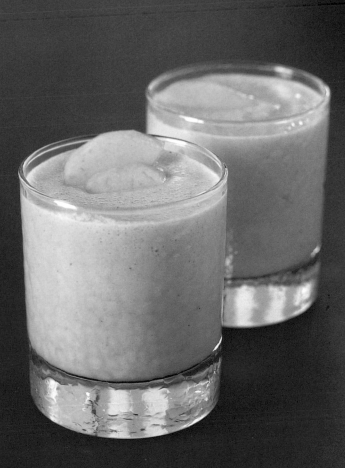

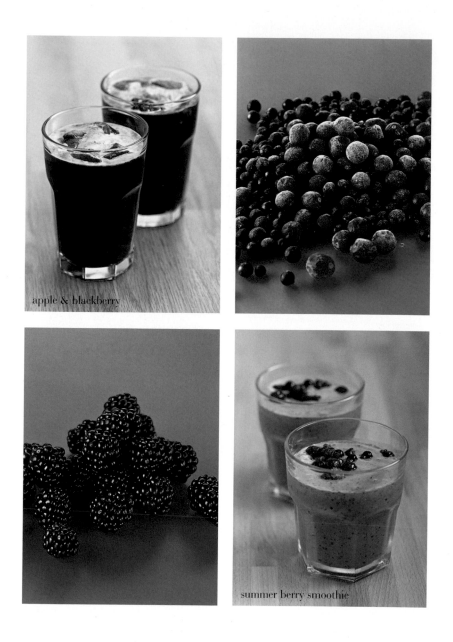

apple & blackberry

summer berry smoothie

apple & blackberry

3 apples
150 g (5 oz) blackberries
300 ml (10 fl oz) water

Juice the fruit then stir in the water. Pour into a glass and add a couple of ice cubes.

makes 600 ml (1 pint)

apple & blueberry smoothie

2 large apples
125 g (4 oz) fresh or frozen
  blueberries

Juice the apple, then whizz in a blender with the blueberries. Serve in a tumbler.

makes 150 ml (5 fl oz)

summer berry smoothie

150 g (5 oz) frozen mixed berries
300 ml (10 fl oz) vanilla-flavoured
  soya milk
1 teaspoon clear honey (optional)

Place the berries, milk and honey, if using, in a blender and process until thick. Serve immediately decorated with berries, if liked.

makes 400 ml (14 fl oz)

apricot smoothie

200 g (7 oz) can apricots in
  natural juice, drained
150 g (5 oz) apricot yogurt
150 ml (5 fl oz) ice-cold
  semi-skimmed milk

Place the apricots, yogurt and milk in a blender and process until smooth. Serve immediately with ice and decorated with slices of apricot, if liked.

makes 400 ml (14 fl oz)

go green

2 carrots
2 celery sticks
100 g (3½ oz) spinach
100 g (3½ oz) lettuce
25 g (1 oz) parsley

Juice the ingredients and whizz in a blender with a couple of ice cubes. Garnish with parsley sprigs, if liked.

makes 200 ml (7 fl oz)

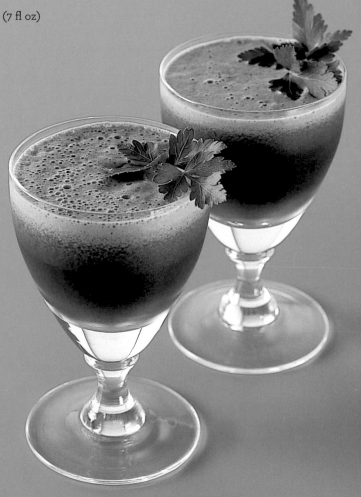

drink your greens

100 g (3½ oz) Brussels sprouts
100 g (3½ oz) carrot
100 g (3½ oz) Jerusalem artichokes
100 g (3½ oz) green beans
100 g (3½ oz) lettuce
½ lemon

Juice all the ingredients. Serve decorated with slivers of green bean and carrot, if liked.

makes 200 ml (7 fl oz)

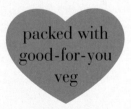

packed with
good-for-you
veg

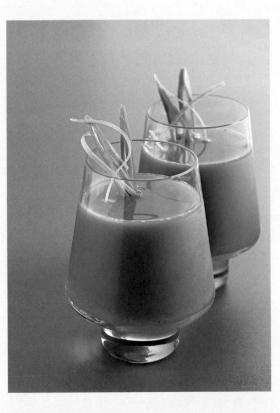

grapefruit, parsnip & sweet potato

½ large grapefruit
1 small parsnip
1 small sweet potato

Juice all the ingredients and blend the juice with an ice cube. Serve over
ice and, if liked, decorate with a sliver of parsnip.

makes 200 ml (7 fl oz)

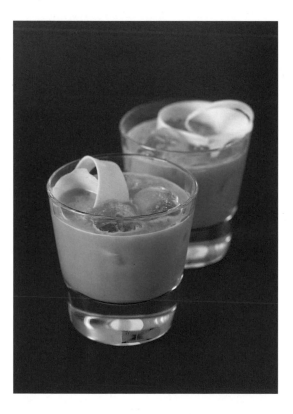

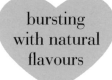
bursting
with natural
flavours

strawberry, kiwifruit & almond smoothie

200 ml (7 fl oz) soya milk
2 kiwifruit
100 g (3½ oz) fresh or frozen strawberries
25 g (1 oz) flaked almonds

Put all the ingredients in a food processor or blender. If using fresh rather than frozen strawberries add a few ice cubes, then process until smooth. Pour into a glass and decorate with flaked almonds, if liked.

makes 300 ml (10 fl oz)

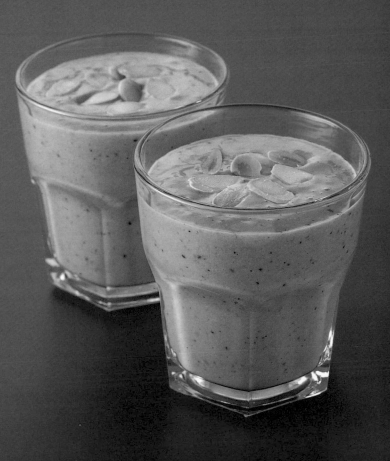

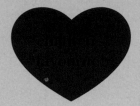

super stripy smoothie

250 g (8 oz) raspberries
200 ml (7 fl oz) apple juice
200 g (7 oz) blueberries
4 tablespoons Greek yogurt
100 ml (3½ fl oz) skimmed milk
1 tablespoon clear honey, or to taste
1 tablespoon wheatgerm (optional)

Purée the raspberries with half of the apple juice. Purée the blueberries with the remaining apple juice. Mix together the yogurt, milk, honey and wheatgerm, if using. Add a spoonful of the raspberry purée.

Pour the blueberry purée into the glass. Pour on the yogurt mixture carefully and finally pour the raspberry purée over the surface of the yogurt. Serve chilled.

makes 200 ml (7 fl oz)

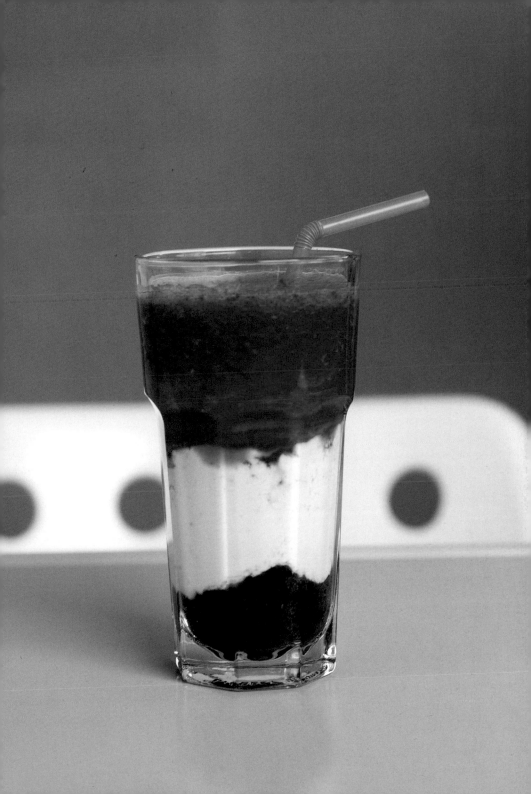

tropical smoothie

1 ripe mango
300 ml (10 fl oz) pineapple juice
rind and juice of ½ lime

Roughly chop the mango flesh and freeze for at least 2 hours or overnight.
Place the frozen mango in a blender with the pineapple juice and lime rind
and juice and process until thick. Decorate with lime wedges, if liked.

makes 400 ml (14 fl oz)

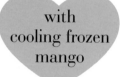

**with
cooling frozen
mango**

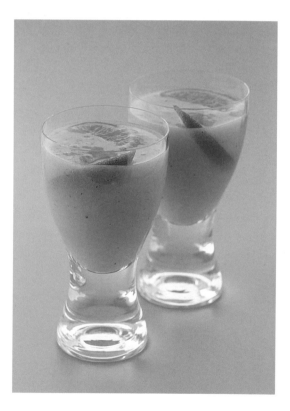

mango lassi

½ large mango
100 ml (3½ fl oz) natural yogurt
100 ml (3½ fl oz) water

Blend the mango flesh with the other ingredients until smooth then serve
decorated with mint.

makes 350 ml (12 fl oz)

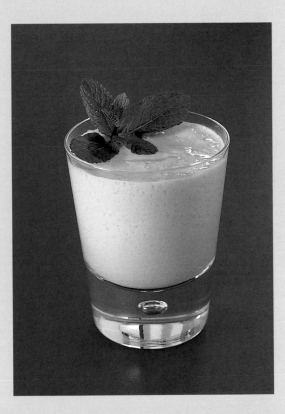

citrus & fig refresher

½ grapefruit
2 fresh figs
½ small orange
½ lemon

Juice all the fruit then blend with an ice cube to chill. Decorate with slices of fig, if liked.

makes 200 ml (7 fl oz)

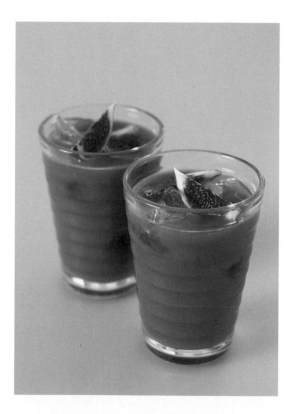

zesty pineapple & avocado smoothie

½ pineapple, about 225 g (7½ oz)
1 lemon
½ large avocado

Juice the pineapple flesh and lemon. Place the juice into a blender with the avocado and process until smooth. Serve with a slice of lemon, if liked.

makes 200 ml (7 fl oz)

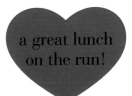

a great lunch
on the run!

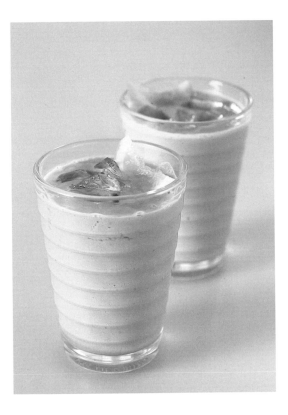

broccoli, carrot & beetroot

250 g (8 oz) broccoli
2 small carrots
1 small beetroot, about 50 g (2 oz)

Juice all the ingredients together and then serve in a tall glass.
Add crushed ice and garnish with a coriander sprig, if liked.

makes 200 ml (7 fl oz)

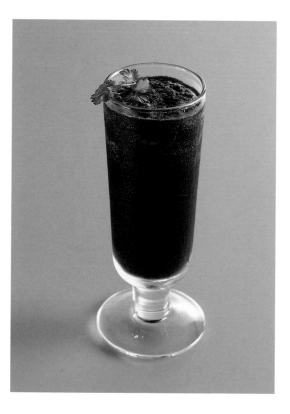

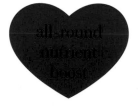

all-round
nutrient
boost

parsnip, fennel & cucumber

1 parsnip
1 fennel bulb
200 g (7 oz) cucumber

Juice all the ingredients and serve over ice with mint, if liked.

makes 200 ml (7 fl oz)

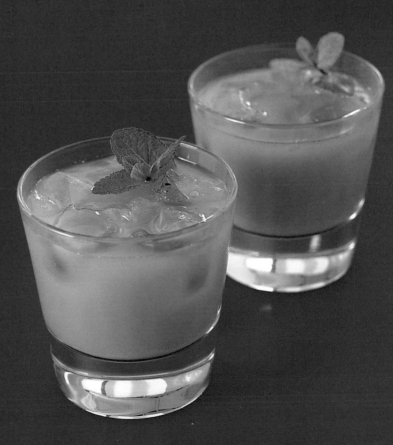

super seven (left)

75 g (3 oz) carrot
50 g (2 oz) green pepper
25 g (1 oz) spinach
25 g (1 oz) onion
50 g (2 oz) celery
75 g (3 oz) cucumber
50 g (2 oz) tomato
sea salt and pepper

Juice the ingredients and season with sea salt and pepper. If liked, decorate with tomato quarters.

makes 200 ml (7 fl oz)

nutritious food, fast

apple, kiwifruit & avocado (right)

250 g (8 oz) apple
50 g (2 oz) celery
50 g (2 oz) kiwifruit
½ lemon
100 g (3½ oz) avocado

Juice the apple, celery, kiwifruit and lemon. Transfer to a blender with the avocado and whizz for 20 seconds. Decorate with kiwifruit slices, if liked.

makes 200 ml (7 fl oz)

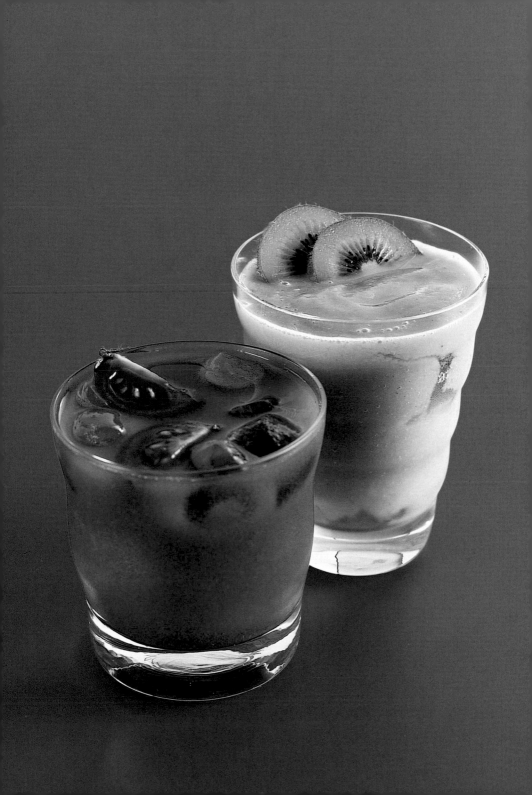

pineapple, celery & lemon

¼ pineapple, about 150 g (5 oz)
3 celery sticks
½ lemon

Juice all the ingredients then serve over ice in a tall glass. Decorate with sprigs of mint, if liked.

makes 200 ml (7 fl oz)

lemon & grape

1 lemon
100 g (3½ oz) green grapes

Juice both ingredients then make up to 200 ml (7 fl oz) with cold water. Serve over ice. If you like, add hot water instead to make a hot toddy.

makes 200 ml (7 fl oz)

papaya, raspberry & grapefruit

½ papaya
150 g (5 oz) raspberries
½ grapefruit

Juice the flesh of the papaya with the grapefruit (pith left on) and the raspberries. Serve with a few ice cubes and, if liked, decorate with lemon slices.

makes 200 ml (7 fl oz)

caribbean smoothie

1 papaya
1 orange
1 banana
300 ml (10 fl oz) apple juice

Whizz the orange, papaya and banana in a blender. Add the mixture to the apple juice and stir well. Serve with ice, if liked.

makes 400 ml (14 fl oz)

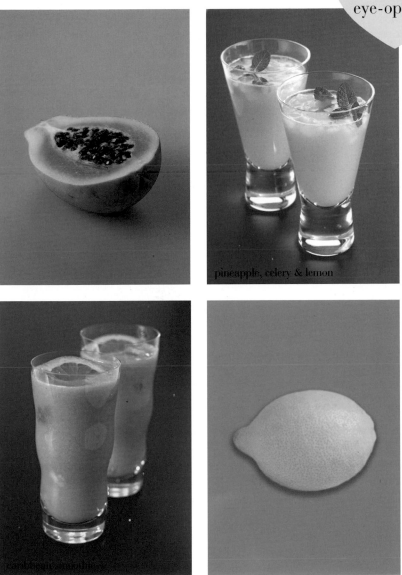

pineapple, celery & lemon

caribbean smoothie

watermelon, pomegranate & raspberry smoothie

¼ watermelon, about 300 g (10 oz) flesh
1 pomegranate
100 g (3½ oz) raspberries

Scoop out the pomegranate seeds, juice with the watermelon and raspberries and serve over ice. Decorate with pomegranate seeds, if liked.

makes 200 ml (7 fl oz)

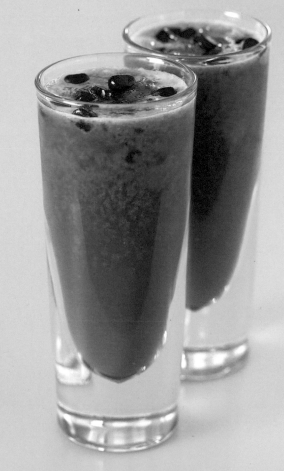

to satisfy a
sweet tooth

celeriac, beetroot & apple

100 g (3½ oz) celeriac, peeled
1 beetroot, about 50 g (2 oz)
1 carrot
50 g (2 oz) radicchio
1 apple

Juice all the ingredients, then process the juice in a blender with a couple of ice cubes. Garnish with slivers of radicchio, if liked.

makes 200 ml (7 fl oz)

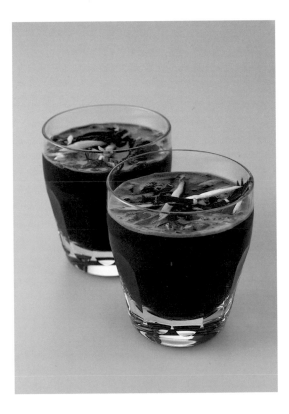

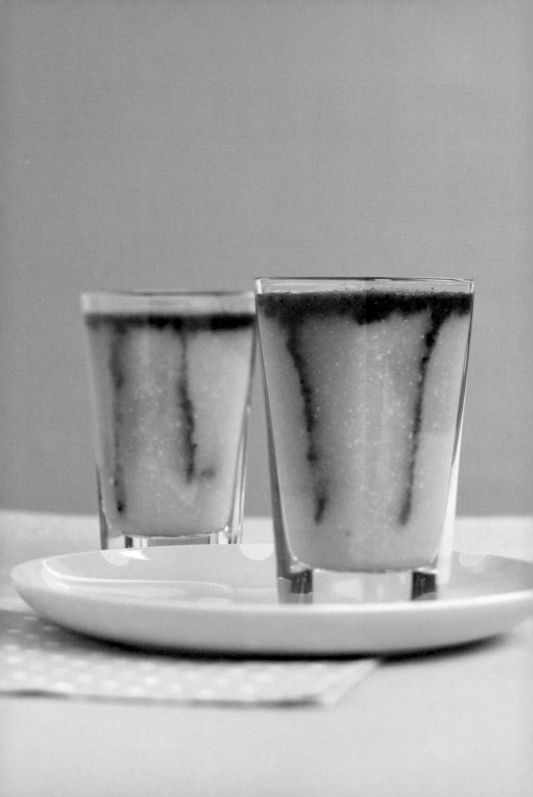

mango & blackcurrant smoothie

3 mangoes
2 tablespoons mango sorbet
100 ml (3½ fl oz) apple juice
200 g (7 oz) blackcurrants or blueberries

Purée the mango with the mango sorbet and half the apple juice. Set aside to chill. Purée the blackcurrants with the rest of the apple juice.

To serve, divide the mango smoothie between two glasses. Place a spoon on the surface of the mango, holding it as flat as you can, and pour on the blackcurrant purée. Drag a teaspoon or skewer down the inside of the glass, to make vertical stripes around the glass.

makes 400 ml (14 fl oz)

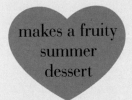

makes a fruity
summer
dessert

strawberry, redcurrant & orange

100 g (3½ oz) strawberries
75 g (3 oz) redcurrants
½ orange
125 ml (4 fl oz) water
½ teaspoon clear honey (optional)

Juice the fruit, then add the water. Pour into a glass, stir in the honey, if using, and add some ice cubes. Decorate with redcurrants, if liked.

makes 250 ml (8 fl oz)

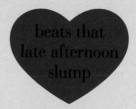
beats that
late afternoon
slump

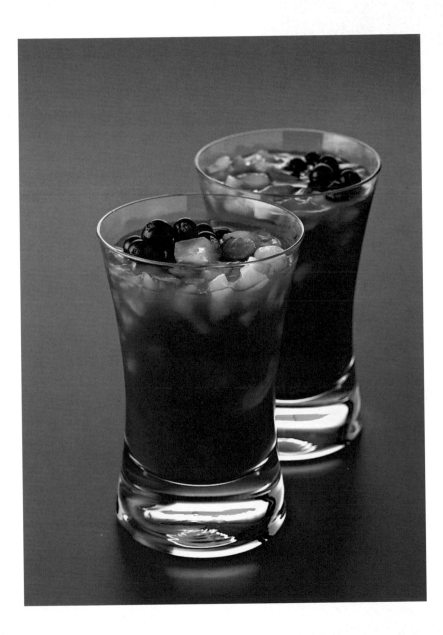

celery, grape & avocado smoothie

2 celery sticks
100 g (3½ oz) green grapes
½ small avocado

Juice the celery and grapes. Put the juice into a blender with the avocado
and serve with a couple of ice cubes and a celery leaf, if liked.

makes 200 ml (7 fl oz)

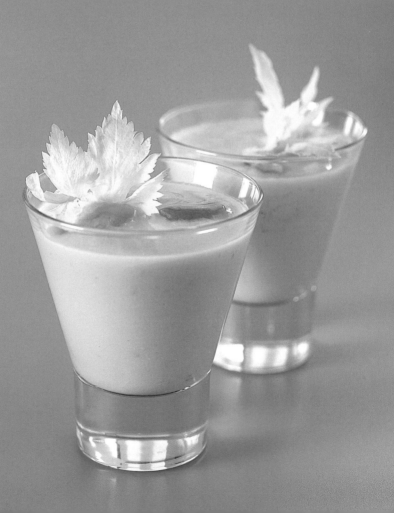

banana, orange & sunflower seed smoothie

1 small banana
juice of 2 large oranges
25 g (1 oz) sunflower seeds
strawberry halves, to serve (optional)

Put the banana, orange juice and sunflower seeds into a blender with a few ice cubes and process until smooth. Serve in a large tumbler and decorate with some strawberry halves, if liked.

makes 300 ml (10 fl oz)

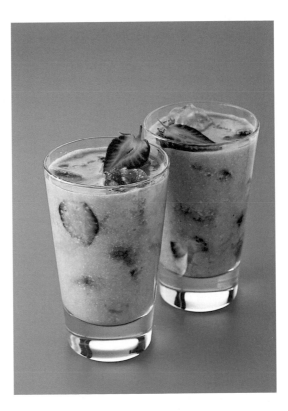

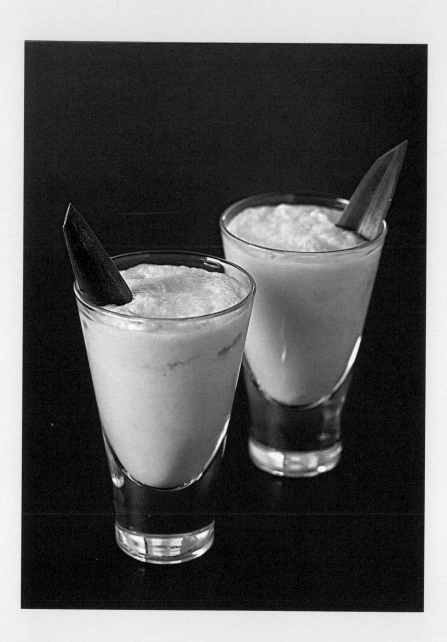

pineapple & coconut smoothie

½ pineapple, about 215 g (7 oz)
100 ml (3½ fl oz) coconut milk
100 ml (3½ fl oz) soya milk

Place all the ingredients in a blender with some ice cubes and blend until the mixture is smooth. Decorate with pineapple leaves, if liked.

makes 300 ml (10 fl oz)

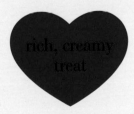

rich, creamy
treat

carrot, radish & apple

2 large carrots
50 g (2 oz) radishes
1 large apple

Juice the carrots, radishes and apple. Pour the juice into a blender and process with a couple of ice cubes. Serve decorated with slices of apple, if liked.

makes 200 ml (7 fl oz)

sweet with a hint of heat

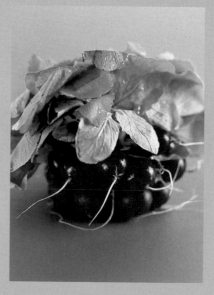

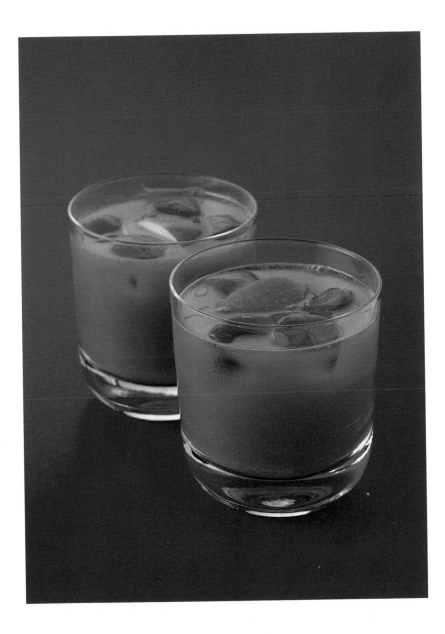

rhubarb & custard smoothie

150 g (5 oz) can rhubarb
150 g (5 oz) carton ready-made custard
100 ml (3½ fl oz) ice-cold semi-skimmed milk
1 teaspoon icing sugar (optional)

Drain the rhubarb then put it into a blender with the custard, milk and icing sugar, if using, and process until smooth. Pour into a glass, add a couple of ice cubes, if liked, and serve immediately.

makes 300 ml (10 fl oz)

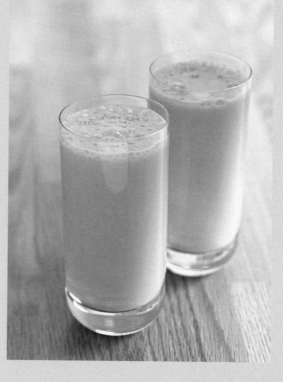

new take on
a traditional
pud

pink grapefruit & lychee smoothie

½ large pink grapefruit
100 g (3½ oz) canned lychees (drained weight)

Juice the grapefruit and place in a blender with the lychees. Blend until
smooth. Pour into a glass and decorate with a slice of grapefruit, if liked.

makes 200 ml (7 fl oz)

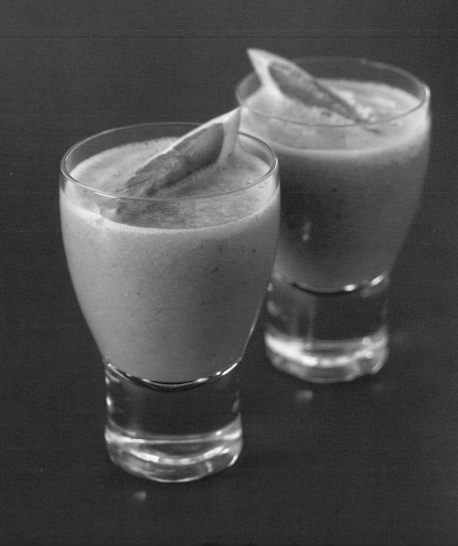

broccoli, apple & cucumber

100 g (3½ oz) broccoli
1 small apple
100 g (3½ oz) cucumber

Juice the broccoli with the apple and cucumber and serve in a tall glass.
Decorate with cucumber slivers, if liked.

makes 200 ml (7 fl oz)

wholesome and
reviving

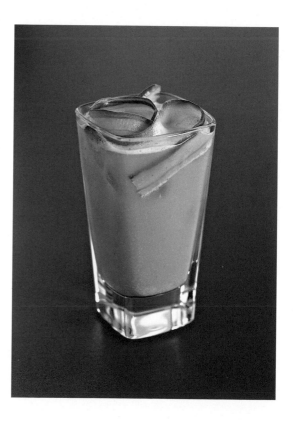

apple, apricot & peach

2 apples
3 apricots
1 peach

Juice the apples, apricots and peach. Pour into a blender with a few ice cubes and whizz for 10 seconds. Serve in a tall glass and decorate with peach slices, if liked.

makes 200 ml (7 fl oz)

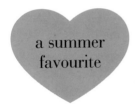

a summer
favourite

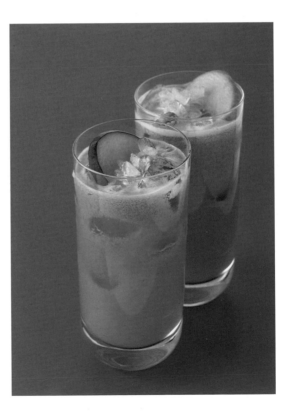

beetroot, strawberry & apple

2 small beetroot, about 100 g (3½ oz)
100 g (3½ oz) strawberries
1 small apple

Juice all the ingredients and serve decorated with a twist of apple peel,
if liked.

makes 300 ml (10 fl oz)

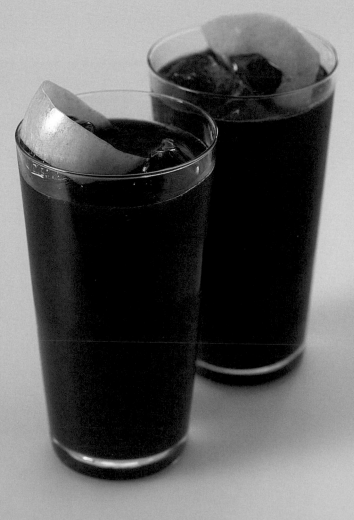

melon, blackberry & kiwifruit

¼ cantaloupe melon
100 g (3½ oz) fresh or frozen blackberries
2 kiwifruit

Juice the melon flesh, blackberries and kiwifruit, then put the juices in
a blender and process with a couple of ice cubes. Pour into a glass and
serve decorated with a few blackberries, if liked.

makes 250 ml (8 fl oz)

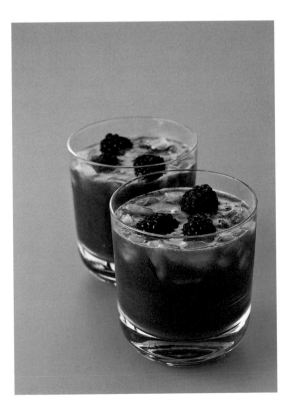

grape, fennel & mango

100 g (3½ oz) green grapes
1 small fennel bulb
½ large mango

Juice the grapes and fennel then put into a blender with the mango and a couple of ice cubes and blend. Serve with fennel fronds, if liked.

makes 300 ml (10 fl oz)

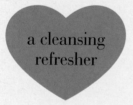

a cleansing
refresher

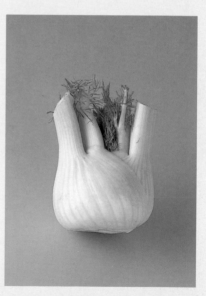

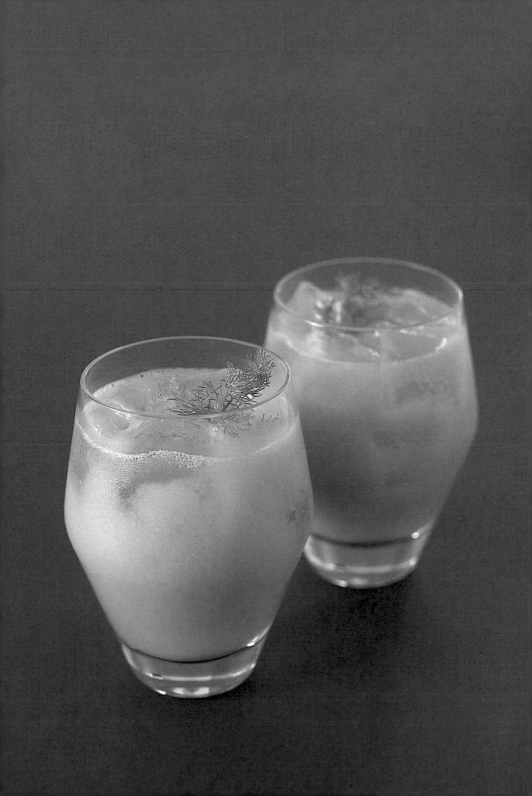

pear & pineapple

2 pears
½ lime
½ pineapple, about 200 g (7 oz)

Juice all the fruit. Then pour into a glass. Add some ice cubes and decorate with wedges of pineapple, if liked.

makes 300 ml (10 fl oz)

blockbuster

25 g (1 oz) each of pineapple, papaya, carrot, sweet potato, apple, cantaloupe melon, grapefruit and celery.

Juice all the ingredients together and serve in a tall glass over ice. Decorate with slices of apple, if liked.

makes 250 ml (8 fl oz)

carrot, cauliflower & tomato

100 g (3½ oz) cauliflower
2 small carrots
1 large tomato

Juice all the ingredients. Stir to mix then serve poured over ice and garnished with carrot tops, if liked.

makes 200 ml (7 fl oz)

grape, lettuce & ginger

200 g (7 oz) green grapes
200 g (7 oz) lettuce
2.5 cm (1 inch) cube fresh root ginger, roughly chopped

Juice all the ingredients. Serve over ice, or pour into a blender and process with ice cubes for a zingy icy slush. Decorate with green or red grapes, if liked.

makes 200 ml (7 fl oz)

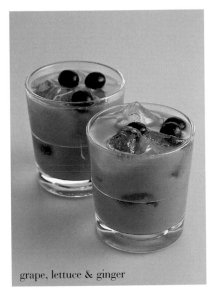

grape, lettuce & ginger

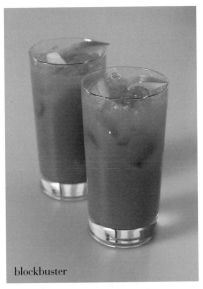

blockbuster

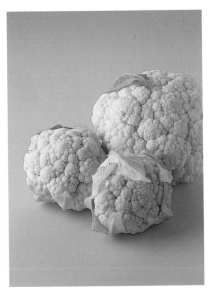

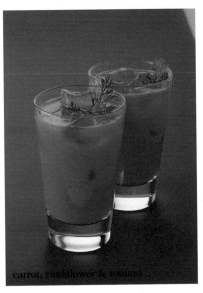

carrot, cauliflower & tomato

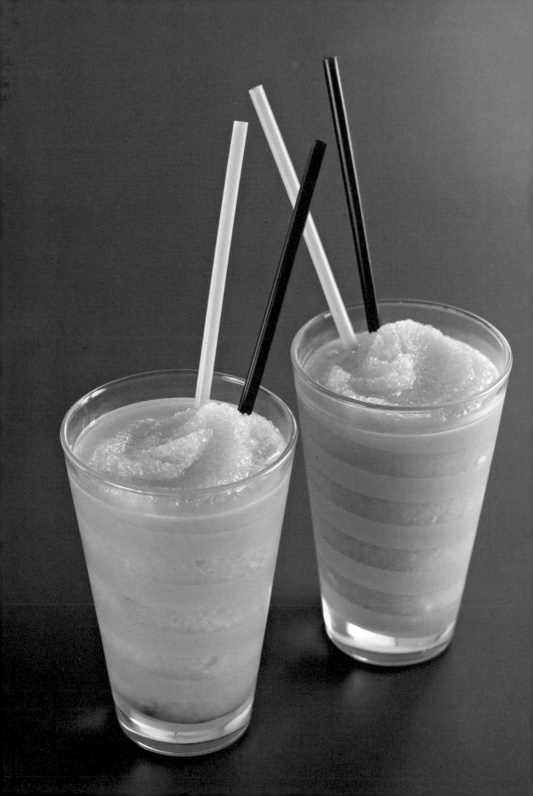

mango & apple slush

½ large mango
2 small apples
juice of ½ lime

Juice the ingredients then blend with a couple of ice cubes to make a fruity slush.

makes 200 ml (7 fl oz)

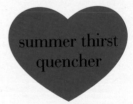

summer thirst quencher

cranberry, banana & sesame smoothie

40 g (1½ oz) dried cranberries
juice of ½ lemon
1 large banana
1 tablespoon sesame seeds
2 tablespoons Greek yogurt
200 ml (7 fl oz) whole or semi-skimmed milk

Process the cranberries and lemon juice in a blender until the berries are finely chopped. Add the banana and sesame seeds then purée, scraping the mixture down from the sides of the bowl if necessary. Add the yogurt and milk, processing until smooth and frothy. Decorate with dried cranberries, if liked.

makes 300 ml (10 fl oz)

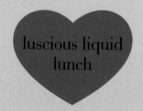
luscious liquid
lunch

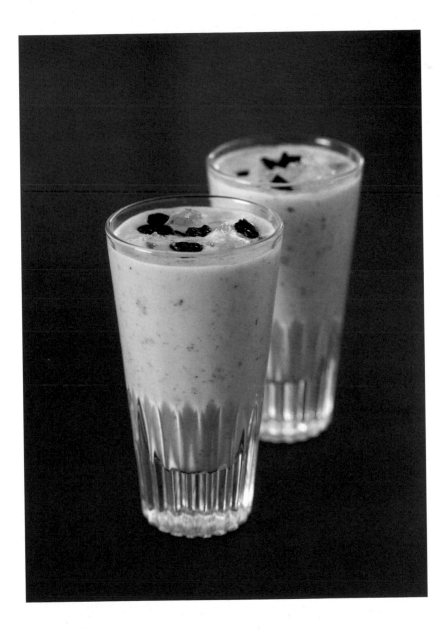

grape, cranberry & cherry smoothie

100 g (3½ oz) green or red grapes
100 ml (3½ fl oz) cranberry juice
100 g (3½ oz) pitted cherries

Juice the grapes then blend with the other ingredients. Serve over ice and decorate with fresh cherries, if liked.

makes 250 ml (8 fl oz)

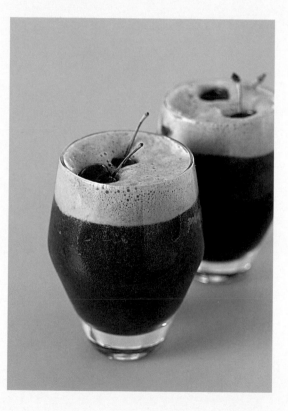

lime, orange & mango

1 lime
2 small oranges
½ large mango

Juice the lime and oranges and whizz in a food processor or blender together with the mango flesh and an ice cube. Decorate with lime slices, if liked.

makes 250 ml (8 fl oz)

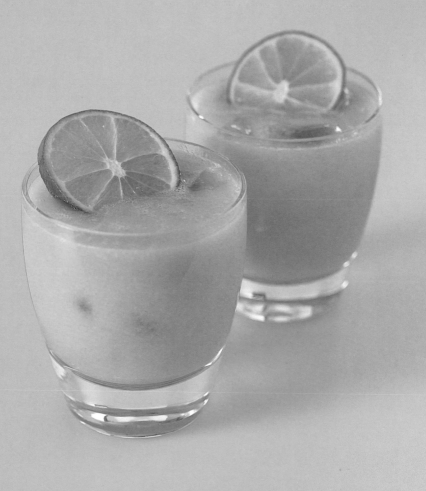

plum punch

1 peach
2 plums
1 kiwifruit

Juice all the ingredients and serve over ice cubes. Decorate with plum slices, if liked.

makes 200 ml (7 fl oz)

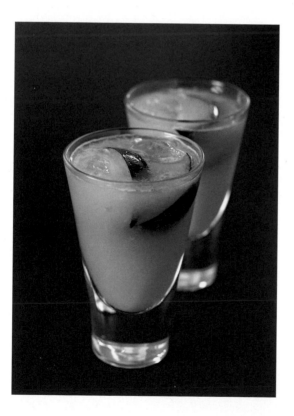

minty pepper & orange

½ red pepper
½ yellow pepper
½ orange pepper
1 orange
1 tablespoon mint leaves

Juice the peppers and orange and serve in a tumbler with ice cubes.
Stir in the mint and decorate with more mint leaves, if liked.

makes 200 ml (7 fl oz)

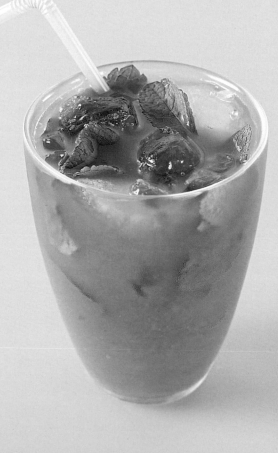

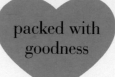

packed with
goodness

traffic light smoothie

3 kiwifruit
150 ml (¼ pint) tangy flavoured yogurt, such as lemon or orange
1 small mango
2 tablespoons orange or apple juice
150 g (5 oz) raspberries
1–2 teaspoons clear honey

Peel the kiwifruit and whizz in a blender until smooth. Spoon the
kiwifruit mixture into two tall glasses. Top each with a spoonful of yogurt,
spreading the yogurt to the sides of the glasses.

Blend the mango to a purée with the orange or apple juice and spoon into
the glasses. Top with another layer of yogurt.

Blend the raspberries and push through a sieve over a bowl to extract the
seeds. Check their sweetness. You might need to stir in a little honey if
they're very sharp. Spoon the raspberry purée into the glasses.

makes 400 ml (14 fl oz)

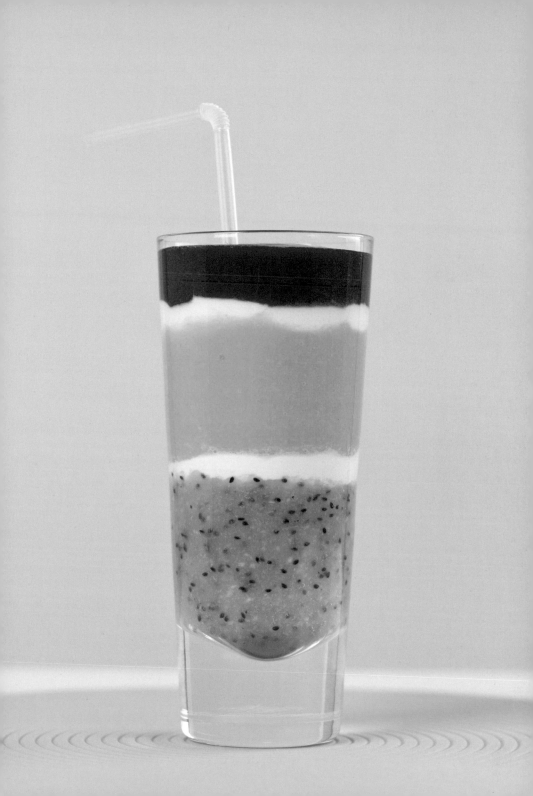

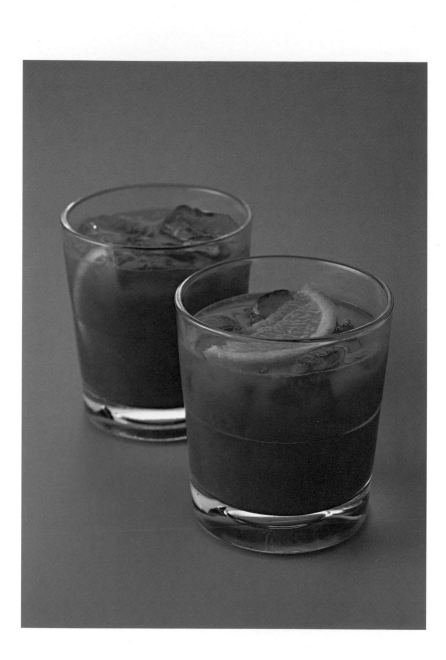

watermelon & orange

¼ watermelon, about 300 g (10 oz) flesh
2 oranges

Juice the fruit, pour it into a glass and add a couple of ice cubes to chill.
Decorate with slices of orange, if liked.

makes 300 ml (10 fl oz)

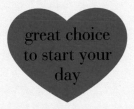

great choice
to start your
day

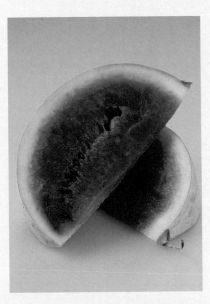

raspberry ripple smoothie

100 g (3½ oz) fresh raspberries
100 g (3½ oz) natural yogurt
100 ml (3½ fl oz) soya milk

Whizz the raspberries, natural yogurt and soya milk together in a blender until smooth. Swirl in a little yogurt to decorate.

makes 300 ml (10 fl oz)

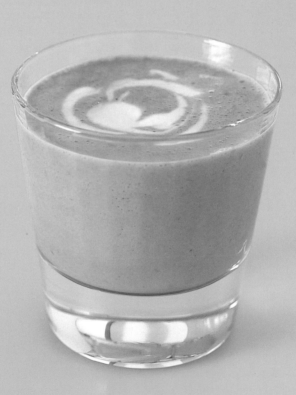

berry, lychee & coconut smoothie

100 g (3½ oz) frozen mixed berries
100 g (3½ oz) canned lychees (drained weight)
100 g (3½ oz) coconut milk
100 ml (3½ fl oz) soya milk

Put all the ingredients in a blender with a couple of ice cubes and blend until smooth.

makes 200 ml (7 fl oz)

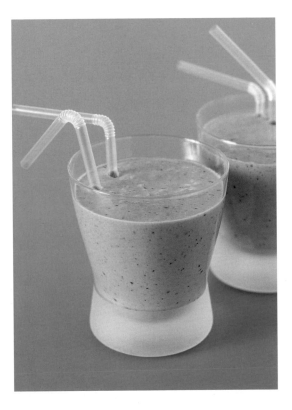

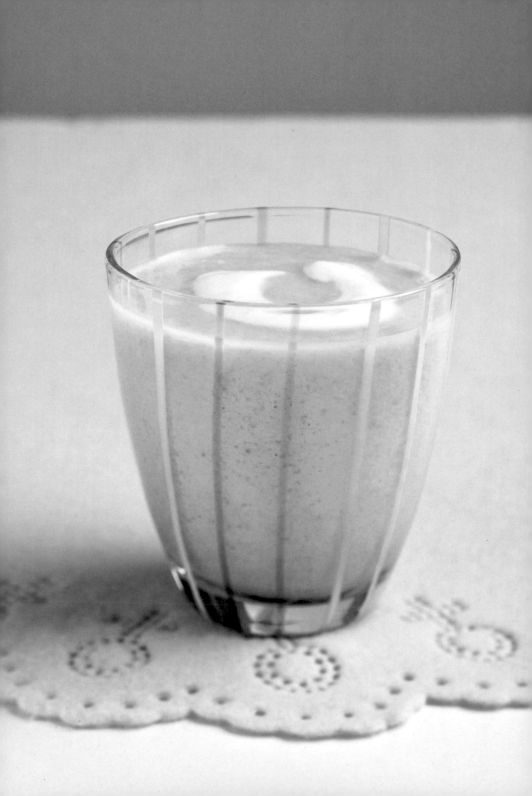

easy peach smoothie

400 g (13 oz) can peaches in natural juice, drained
150 ml (¼ pint) peach or apricot yogurt
200 ml (7 fl oz) orange juice
a little honey (optional)

Place the peaches in a blender with the yogurt, orange juice and honey, if
using, and whizz until smooth. Add a couple of ice cubes, if liked, and top
with a swirl of any remaining yogurt.

makes 400 ml (14 fl oz)

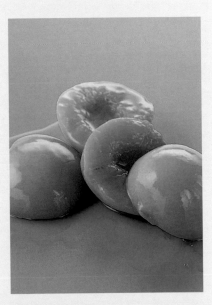

healthy

Wholesome and invigorating, juices and smoothies are the ultimate health drink. A diet that is high in a variety of fruit and vegetables can both prevent and help to cure a wide range of ailments. In this chapter you will find recipes that will become your secret weapon against everything from sinusitis, stress and skin disorders to bloating, morning sickness and arthritis.

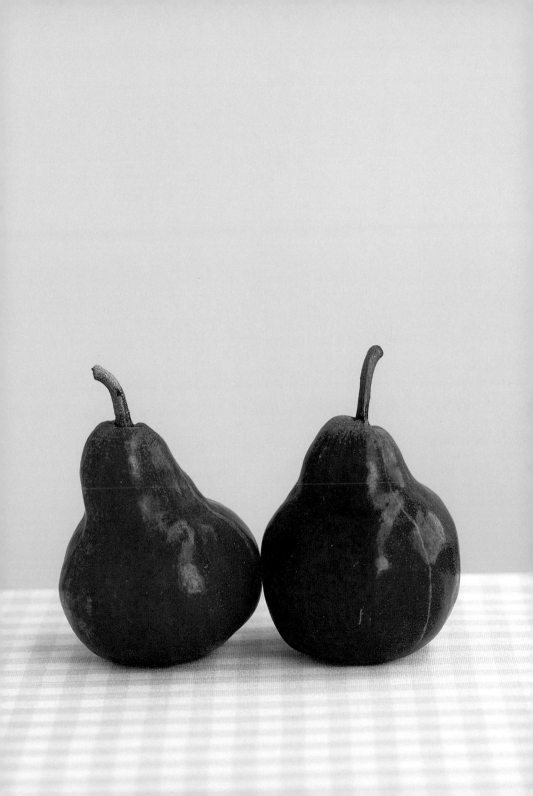

strawberry sunrise

200 g (7 oz) strawberries
2 oranges

Juice the strawberries and oranges. Serve straight over ice, or whizz in a blender with a couple of ice cubes to make a cooling smoothie. Decorate with sliced strawberries, if liked.

makes 200 ml (7 fl oz)

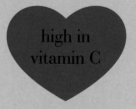

high in
vitamin C

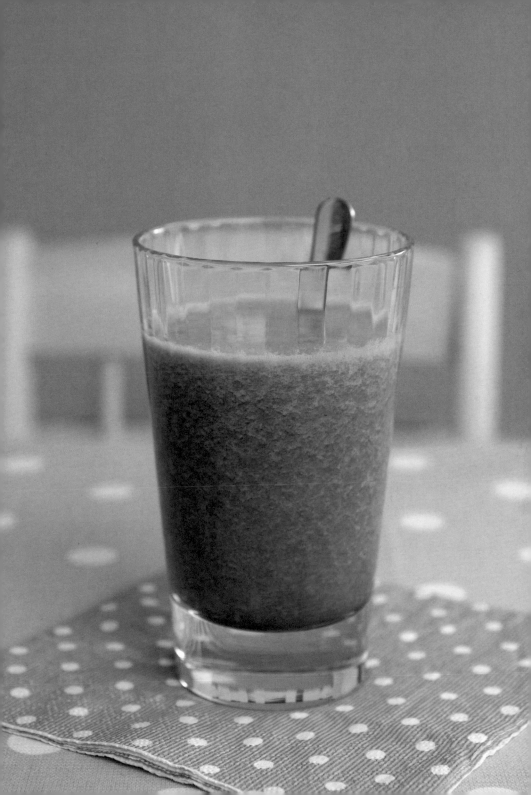

carrot, beetroot & sweet potato

175 g (6 oz) carrot
100 g (3½ oz) beetroot
175 g (6 oz) sweet potato or yam
125 g (4 oz) fennel

Juice all the ingredients. Mix well and serve in a glass with ice cubes.
Decorate with fennel fronds, if liked.

makes 400 ml (14 fl oz)

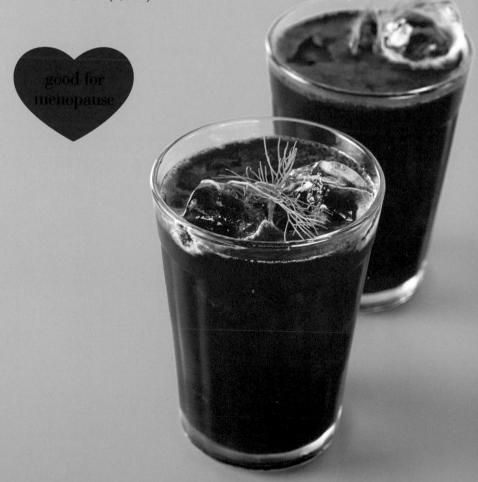

good for
menopause

banana, strawberry & orange smoothie

1 small ripe banana
75 g (3 oz) strawberries
250 ml (8 fl oz) orange juice

Slice the banana and roughly chop the strawberries. Freeze the fruit for at least 2 hours or overnight. Place the frozen fruit and the orange juice in a blender and process until thick. Decorate with strawberries, if liked.

makes 400 ml (14 fl oz)

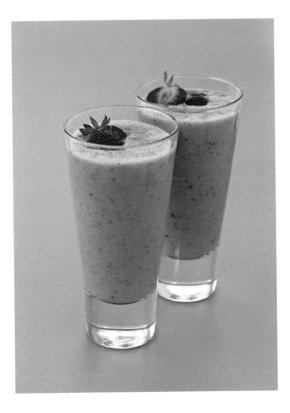

great mood booster

celery, tomato & parsley

2 celery sticks
4 tomatoes
large handful of parsley
zest and juice of ½ lemon

Feed the ingredients into the juicer in alternating batches, along with the lemon juice and zest. Pour the juice into a glass and add a couple of ice cubes

makes 300 ml (10 fl oz)

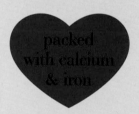

packed
with calcium
& iron

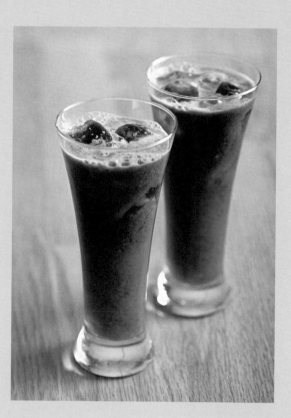

carrot, apple & pink grapefruit

2 carrots
2 apples
1 pink grapefruit
400 ml (14 fl oz) water

Peel the grapefruit and divide into segments. Juice the carrots, apple and grapefruit then add the water. Pour the juice into a glass and add a couple of ice cubes. Decorate with apple slices, if desired.

makes 700 ml (1¼ pints)

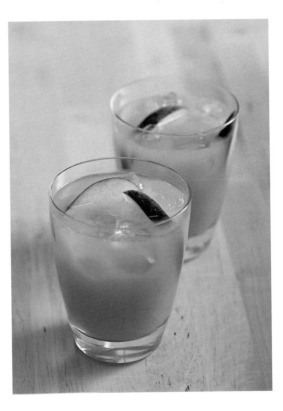

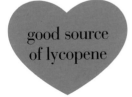

good source of lycopene

melon, cucumber & avocado

175 g (6 oz) cantaloupe melon melon
   (½ large melon)
125 g (4 oz) cucumber
125 g (4 oz) avocado
50 g (2 oz) dried apricots
1 tablespoon wheatgerm

Juice the melon and cucumber. Whizz in a blender with the avocado, apricots, wheatgerm and a couple of ice cubes. Decorate with dried apricot slivers, if liked.

makes 200 ml (7 fl oz)

good for
low fertility

apple, beetroot & celery

200 g (7 oz) apple
50 g (2 oz) beetroot
90 g (3 oz) celery

Juice together all the ingredients and serve over ice in a tumbler.
Decorate with apple slices, if liked.

makes 150 ml (5 fl oz)

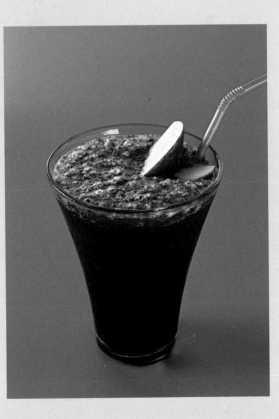

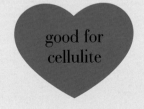

good for
cellulite

orange & apricot

300 g (10 oz) apricots
1 large orange
300 ml (10 fl oz) water

Juice the fruit then add the water.
Serve with ice, if desired.

makes 600 ml (1 pint)

pear, cabbage & celery

250 g (8 oz) pear
125 g (4 oz) cabbage
50 g (2 oz) celery
25 g (1 oz) watercress

Juice all the ingredients and serve
over ice, decorated with celery
sticks, if liked.

makes 200 ml (7 fl oz)

apricot, orange & ginger smoothie

65 g (2½ oz) ready-to-eat apricots
350 ml (12 fl oz) orange juice
3 tablespoons Greek yogurt
4 pieces stem ginger in syrup,
    drained

Roughly chop the apricots and
place in a bowl. Pour over the
orange juice, cover and allow to
stand overnight. Put the mixture
in a blender, add the yogurt and
ginger and process until smooth.
Good source of iron and fibre.

makes 400 ml (14 fl oz)

chamomile, fennel & lemon

1 small fennel bulb
1 lemon
100 ml (3½ fl oz) chilled
    chamomile tea

Juice the fennel and lemon, then
mix with the chamomile tea. Serve
over ice with some lemon slices,
if liked. Good for insomnia.

makes 200 ml (7 fl oz)

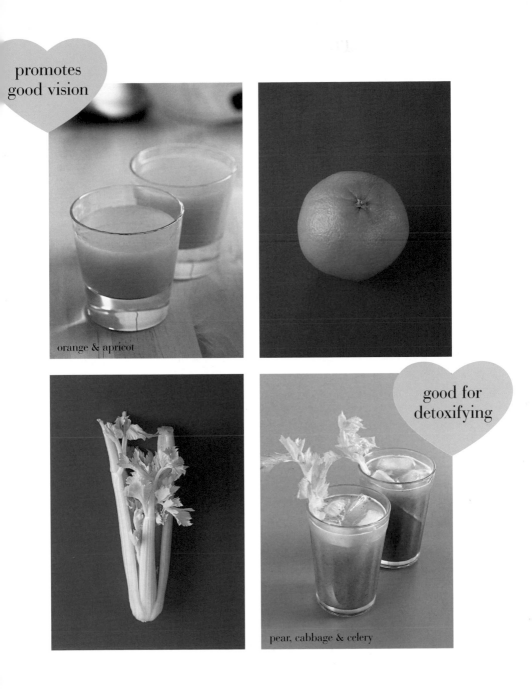

promotes
good vision

orange & apricot

good for
detoxifying

pear, cabbage & celery

orange, cranberry & mango

125 g (4 oz) cranberries
1 mango
1 orange
125 ml (4 fl oz) water
1 teaspoon clear honey

Peel the orange and divide the flesh into segments. Juice the fruit, pour into a glass, and stir in the water and honey. Add a couple of ice cubes and serve immediately. Decorate with cranberries, if desired.

makes 400 ml (14 fl oz)

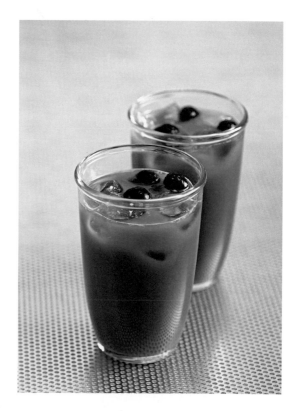

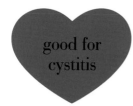

good for
cystitis

cranberry & mango smoothie

1 ripe mango
175 ml (6 fl oz) cranberry juice
150 g (5 oz) Greek yogurt

Place the mango flesh in a blender with the cranberry juice and yogurt and whizz until smooth. Serve immediately with ice and decorated with slices of mango, if desired.

makes 400 ml (14 fl oz)

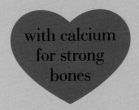

with calcium
for strong
bones

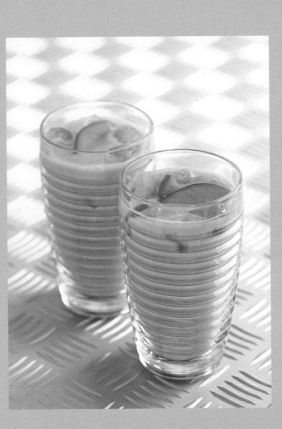

broccoli, kale & celery

100 g (3½ oz) broccoli
100 g (3½ oz) kale
25 g (1 oz) parsley
200 g (7 oz) apple
50 g (2 oz) celery

Juice all the ingredients and serve in a glass over ice. Decorate with kale, if liked.

makes 200 ml (7 fl oz)

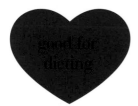

good for
dieting

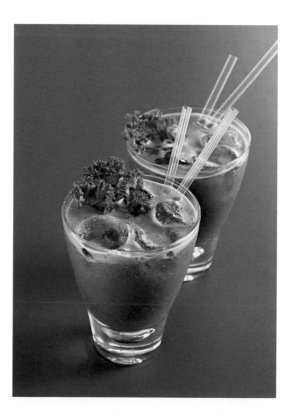

pineapple, grape & lettuce

125 g (4 oz) pineapple
125 g (4 oz) grapes
50 g (2 oz) lettuce
50 g (2 oz) celery

Juice all the ingredients and serve in a tall glass over ice.
Decorate with lettuce leaves, if liked.

makes 200 ml (7 fl oz)

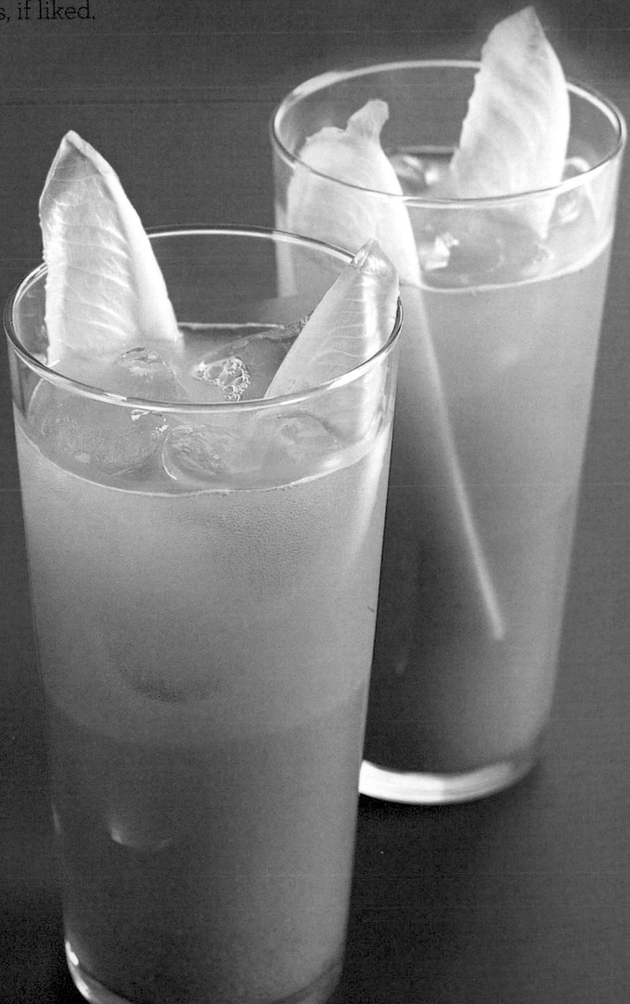

good for
insomnia

celery, fennel & lettuce

50 g (2 oz) celery
50 g (2 oz) fennel
125 g (4 oz) Romaine lettuce
175 g (6 oz) pineapple
1 teaspoon chopped tarragon

Juice all the ingredients and whizz in
a blender with 2 ice cubes. Serve in
a tall glass and decorate with tarragon
sprigs, if liked.

makes 200 ml (7 fl oz)

combats
stress

cranberry & apple smoothie

250 g (8 oz) apple
100 g (3½ oz) frozen cranberries
100 g (3½ oz) live natural yogurt
1 tablespoon clear honey

Juice the apple and whizz in a blender with the other ingredients. Serve in a tumbler over ice cubes.

makes 200 ml (7 fl oz)

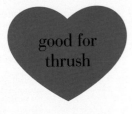

good for thrush

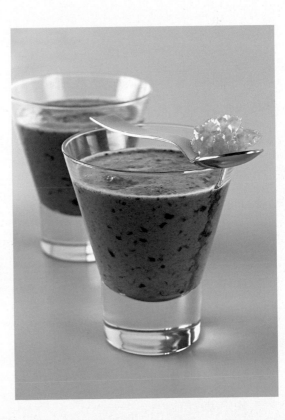

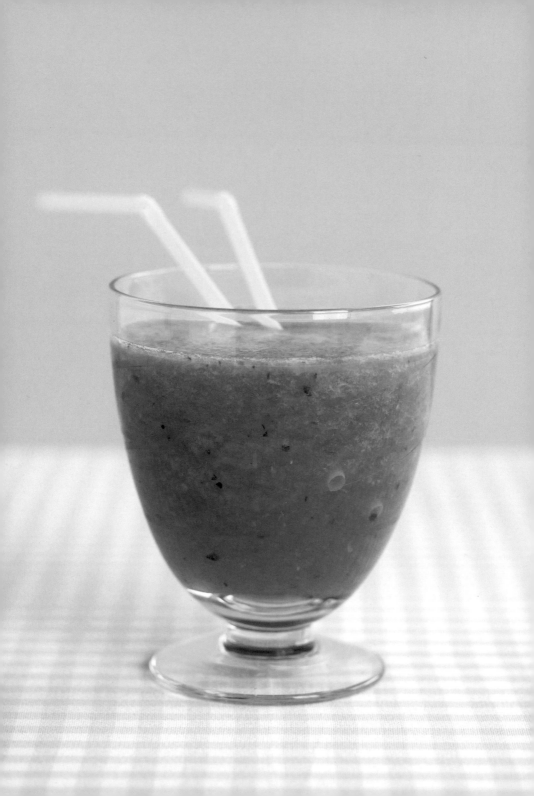

golden wonder

3 apricots
1 large nectarine or peach
2 passion fruit
150 ml (5 fl oz) freshly pressed apple juice

Cut the passion fruit in half, scoop out the pulp and strain through a sieve
to remove the seeds. Put the passion fruit and remaining ingredients in a
blender with a couple of ice cubes and whizz until smooth.

makes 400 ml (14 fl oz)

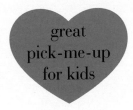

great
pick-me-up
for kids

mango, cranberry & peach smoothie

1 ripe mango
200 ml (7 fl oz) cranberry juice
150 g (5 oz) peach yogurt

Roughly chop the mango flesh and place in a blender with the cranberry juice and yogurt. Process until smooth and pour into a glass. Add a couple of ice cubes and decorate with fresh cranberries, if liked.

makes 400 ml (14 fl oz)

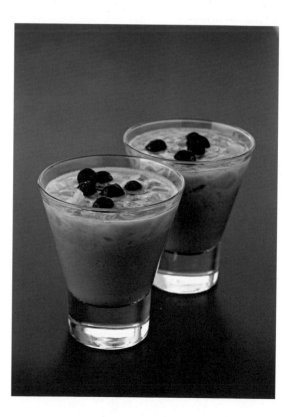

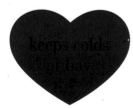

keeps colds
at bay

pink grapefruit, papaya & raspberry

150 g (5 oz) pink grapefruit
150 g (5 oz) papaya
150 g (5 oz) raspberries
½ lime

Scoop out the flesh of the papaya, and juice it with the grapefruit (with the pith left on), and the raspberries. Squeeze in the lime juice and mix. Serve with a few ice cubes and, if liked, decorate with lime slices.

makes 200 ml (7 fl oz)

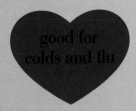

good for colds and flu

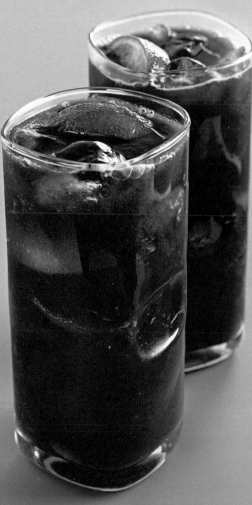

strawberry & pineapple smoothie

150 g (5 oz) strawberries
150 ml (5 fl oz) pineapple juice
150 g (5 oz) strawberry yogurt

Wash, hull and roughly chop the strawberries, then place them in a freezer container and freeze for at least 2 hours or overnight. Place the frozen strawberries, pineapple juice and yogurt in a blender and process until smooth. Serve immediately with ice and decorated with strawberries, if liked.

makes 400 ml (14 fl oz)

prune, apple & cinnamon smoothie

65 g (2½ oz) ready-to-eat prunes
pinch of ground cinnamon
350ml (12 fl oz) apple juice
3 tablespoons Greek yogurt

Roughly chop the prunes into small pieces. Put the prunes and cinnamon in a large bowl. Pour over the apple juice, cover and allow to stand overnight. Place the prunes, apple juice, and yogurt in a blender and process until smooth. Pour into a glass, add ice cubes, sprinkle with cinnamon, and serve immediately.

makes 400 ml (14 fl oz)

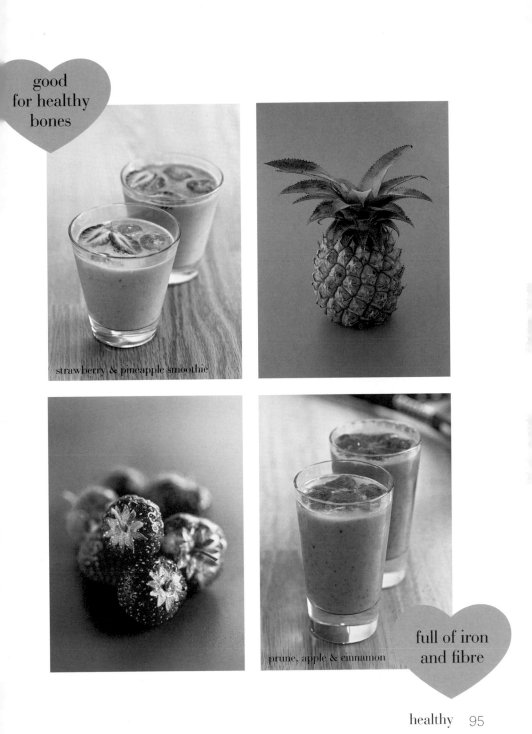

good
for healthy
bones

strawberry & pineapple smoothie

prune, apple & cinnamon

full of iron
and fibre

healthy 95

purple passion

250 g (8 oz) blueberries
125 g (4 oz) grapefruit
250 g (8 oz) apple
2.5 cm (1 inch) cube fresh root ginger, roughly chopped

Juice all the ingredients and serve in a tall glass with ice cubes. Decorate with thin slices of ginger, if liked.

makes 200 ml (7 fl oz)

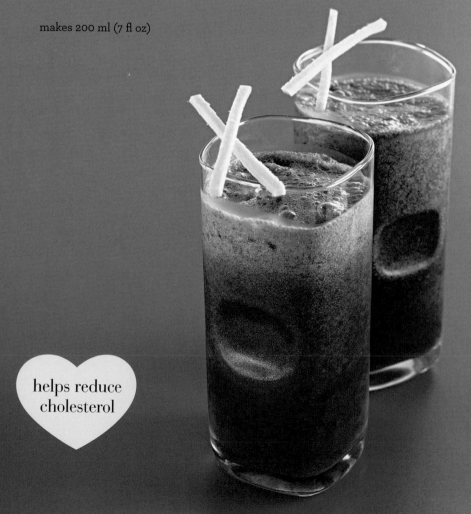

helps reduce
cholesterol

carrot, red cabbage & apple

175 g (6 oz) carrot
250 g (8 oz) apple
125 g (4 oz) red cabbage

Juice all the ingredients, including the apple core. Serve over ice in a tall glass and decorate with slivers of red cabbage, if liked.

makes 150 ml (5 fl oz)

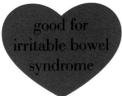

good for
irritable bowel
syndrome

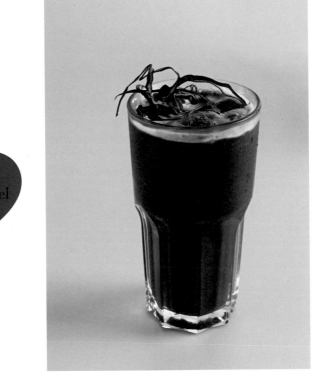

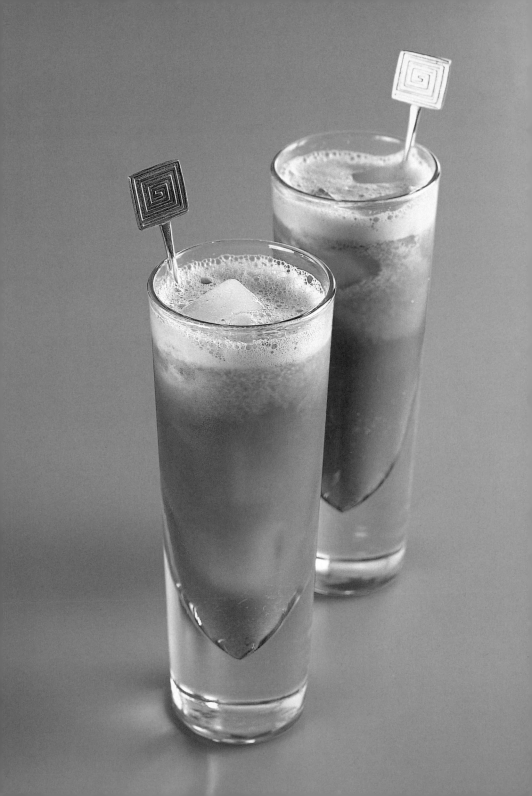

asparagus, dandelion & pear

125 g (4 oz) asparagus spears
10 dandelion leaves
125 g (4 oz) melon
175 g (6 oz) cucumber
200 g (7 oz) pear

Trim the woody bits off the asparagus spears. Roll the dandelion leaves
into a ball and juice them (if you have picked wild leaves, wash them first)
with the asparagus. Peel and juice the melon. Juice the cucumber and pear
with their skins. Whizz everything in a blender and serve in a tall glass
with ice cubes.

makes 200 ml (7 fl oz)

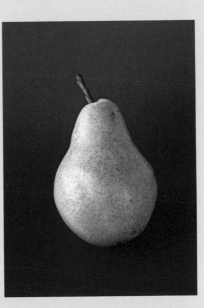

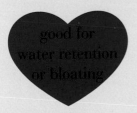

good for
water retention
or bloating

carrot, fig & banana smoothie

250 g (8 oz) carrot
100 g (3½ oz) figs
1 orange
2.5 cm (1 inch) cube fresh root ginger, roughly chopped
100 g (3½ oz) banana

Juice the carrot, figs, orange and ginger. Put the juice into a blender with the banana and two ice cubes and whizz for 20 seconds for a delicious smoothie. Add more ice cubes and decorate with sliced figs, if liked.

makes 200 ml (7 fl oz)

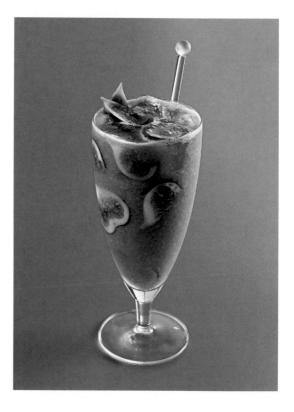

good for
seasonal affective
disorder

root veg

175 g (6 oz) carrot
175 g (6 oz) parsnip
175 g (6 oz) celery
175 g (6 oz) sweet potato
handful of parsley
1 garlic clove

Juice all the ingredients together and whizz in a blender with two ice cubes. Serve in a wide glass decorated with a wedge of lemon and a parsley sprig, if liked.

makes 200 ml (7 fl oz)

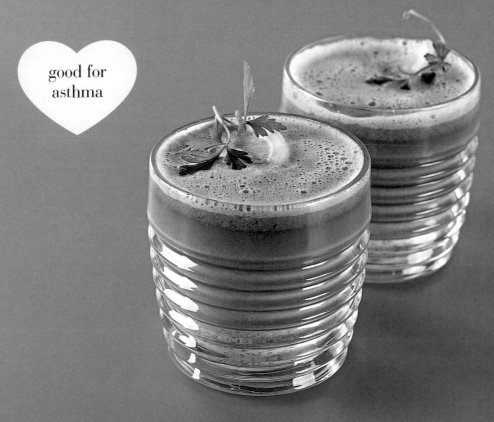

good for
asthma

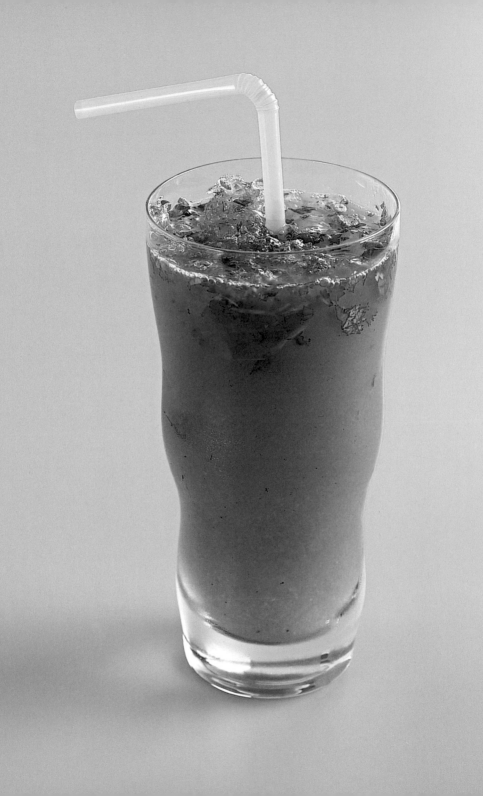

spicy carrot & pineapple

250 g (8 oz) carrot
½ small deseeded chilli or a sprinkling of chilli powder
250 g (8 oz) pineapple
½ lime
1 tablespoon chopped coriander leaves

Juice the carrot, chilli and pineapple. Serve in a tall glass over ice cubes.
Squeeze in the lime juice and stir in the chopped coriander leaves to serve.

makes 200 ml (7 fl oz)

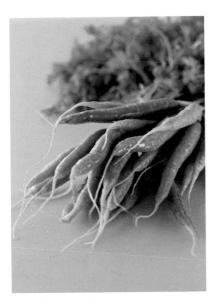

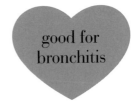

good for
bronchitis

horseradish & lemon (left)

1½ teaspoons pulverized horseradish
½ lemon

Pulverize the horseradish by juicing a small amount and mixing the juice and the pulp. Put it into a shot glass and stir in the lemon juice. Take twice a day.

makes 50 ml (2 fl oz)

good for
sinusitis

carrot, radish & ginger (right)

175 g (6 oz) carrot
100 g (3½ oz) radishes, with tops and leaves
2.5 cm (1 inch) cube fresh root ginger, roughly chopped (optional)

Juice the carrot, radishes and ginger, if using. Add some ice cubes.

makes 200 ml (7 fl oz)

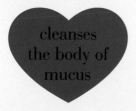

cleanses
the body of
mucus

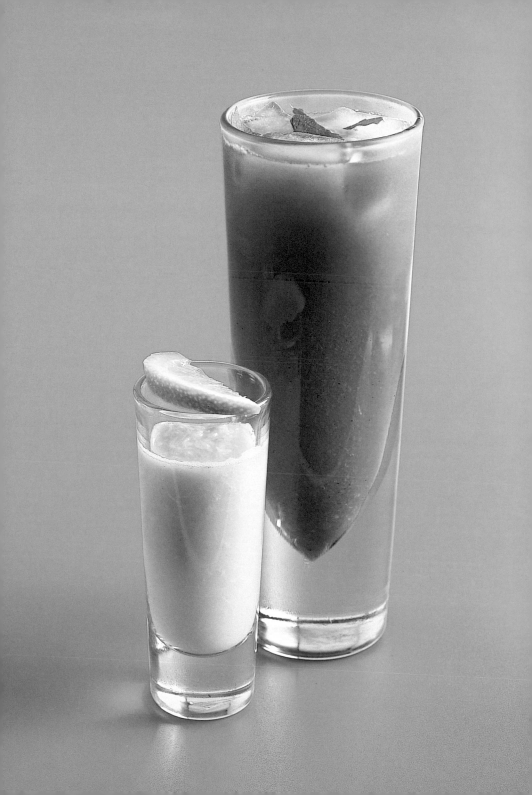

lettuce & fennel

175 g (6 oz) lettuce
125 g (4 oz) fennel
½ lemon

Juice the lettuce, fennel and lemon
and serve on ice. Decorate with
lemon slivers and lettuce leaves,
if liked.

makes 150 ml (5 fl oz)

pear & watercress

250 g (8 oz) pear
125 g (4 oz) watercress
½ lemon

Juice the ingredients and serve
over ice. Add a twist of lemon,
if liked. Good for the digestive
system.

makes 50 ml (2 fl oz)

spinach, parsley & carrot

250 g (8 oz) spinach
25 g (1 oz) parsley
250 g (8 oz) carrot
1 teaspoon spirulina

Juice the spinach, parsley and
carrot and stir in the spirulina.
Serve in a tumbler, decorated with
carrot slivers if liked. Good for
anaemia.

makes 200 ml (7 fl oz)

kiwifruit & cucumber

250 g (8 oz) kiwifruit
125 g (4 oz) cucumber
1 tablespoon pomegranate seeds
   (optional)

Juice the kiwifruit and cucumber
and stir in a tablespoon of
pomegranate seeds, if liked. Serve
with a slice of lime, if liked.

makes 150 ml (5 fl oz)

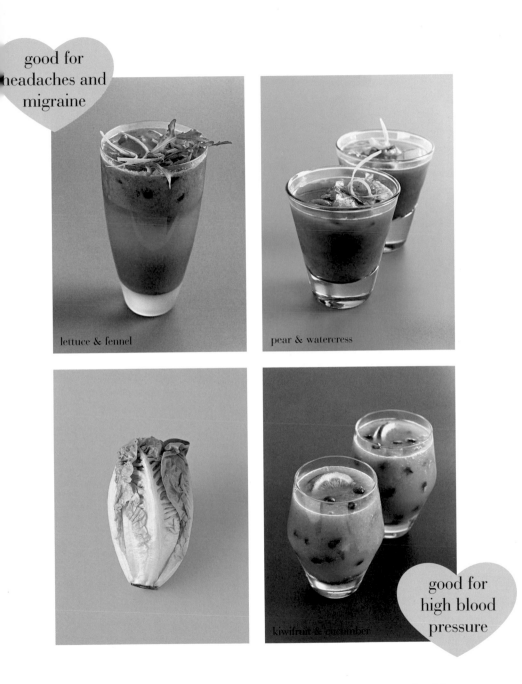

good for
headaches and
migraine

lettuce & fennel

pear & watercress

kiwifruit & cucumber

good for
high blood
pressure

peach & banana smoothie

1 small ripe peach
1 small ripe banana
250 ml (8 fl oz) skimmed milk

Place the peach, banana and milk in a blender and whizz until smooth.
Pour into a glass, add a couple of ice cubes, decorate with a pineapple
wedge, if liked, and serve immediately.

makes 300 ml (10 fl oz)

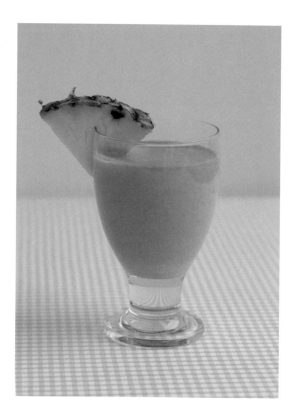

aids
recuperation

blackberry & pineapple

375 g (12 oz) blackberries
1 small pineapple about 375 g (12 oz)

Juice the blackberries first, then the pineapple, to push through the
pulp. Blend the juice with a couple of ice cubes and serve in a tall glass,
decorated with a pineapple sliver, if liked.

makes 200 ml (7 fl oz)

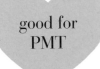

good for
PMT

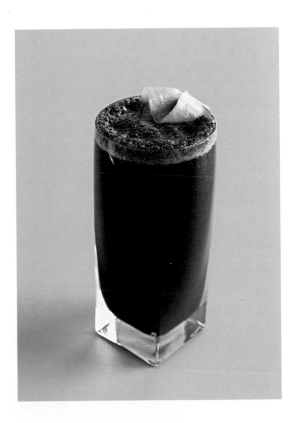

beetroot, onion & carrot

125 g (4 oz) beetroot
125 g (4 oz) watercress
125 g (4 oz) red onion
250 g (8 oz) carrot
1 garlic clove

Juice the ingredients and serve in a tall glass. Decorate with beetroot leaves and watercress, if liked.

makes 200 ml (7 fl oz)

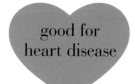

good for
heart disease

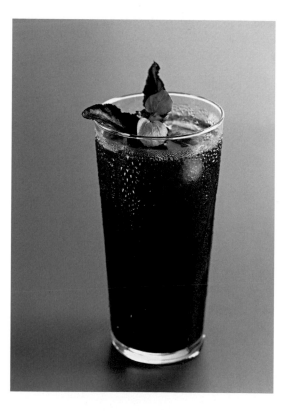

turnip, dandelion & apple

125 g (4 oz) turnips, including the tops
125 g (4 oz) carrot
125 g (4 oz) broccoli
handful of dandelion leaves
175 g (6 oz) apple

Juice all the ingredients and whizz in a blender with a couple of ice cubes.
Serve in a tall glass decorated with dandelion leaves, if liked.

makes 200 ml (7 fl oz)

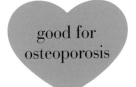

good for
osteoporosis

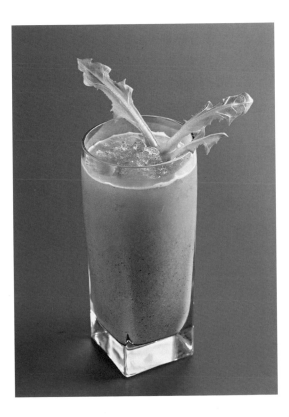

peach fizz

250 g (8 oz) peach
2.5 cm (1 inch) cube fresh root ginger, roughly chopped
sparkling mineral water
mint leaves

Juice the peach and ginger and serve in a tall glass over ice, with a splash of sparkling water and a couple of mint leaves. Sip slowly to calm your stomach.

makes 200 ml (7 fl oz)

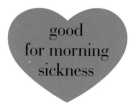

good
for morning
sickness

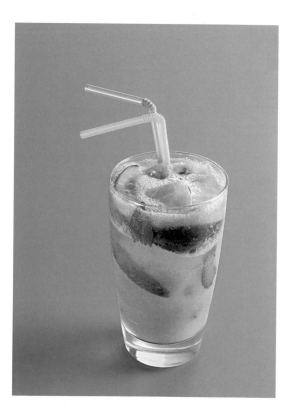

papaya, orange & cucumber

125 g (4 oz) papaya
2 oranges
125 g (4 oz) cucumber

Juice all the ingredients and serve in a tall glass over ice. Decorate with slices of cucumber and papaya, if liked.

makes 200 ml (7 fl oz)

good for
hangovers

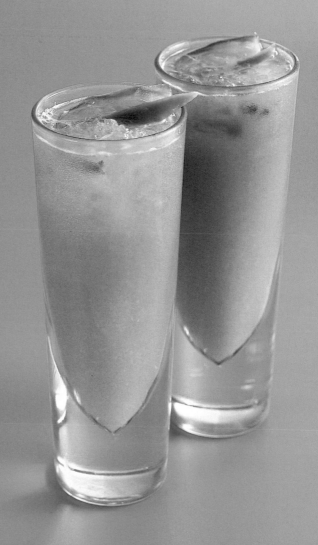

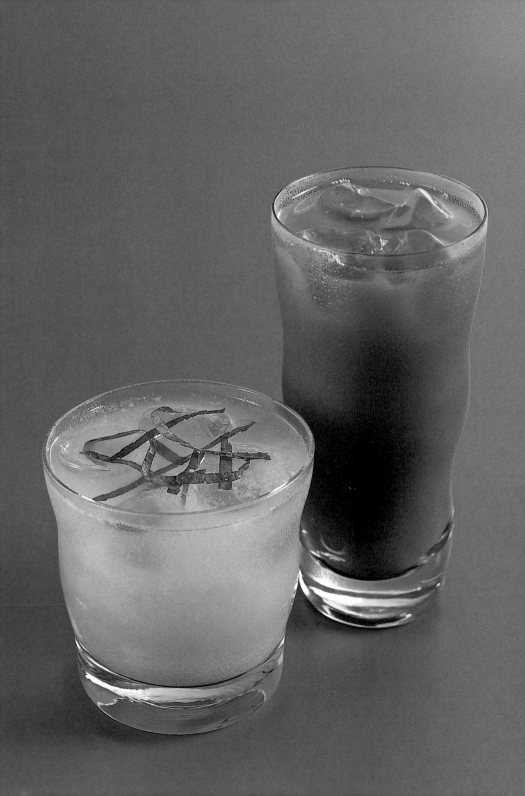

apple & ginger (left)

250 g (8 oz) apple
2.5 cm (1 inch) cube fresh root ginger,
  roughly chopped

Juice the apple and ginger and serve in a glass over ice. Decorate with some chopped mint, if liked. This drink can be diluted with sparkling mineral water to taste.

makes 100 ml (3½ fl oz)

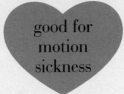

good for
motion
sickness

carrot & cabbage (right)

250 g (8 oz) carrot
250 g (8 oz) green cabbage

Juice the vegetables and serve in a tall glass over ice.

makes 200 ml (7 fl oz)

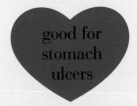

good for
stomach
ulcers

summer smoothie

100 g (3½ oz) pineapple
100 g (3½ oz) grapes
100 g (3½ oz) orange
100 g (3½ oz) apple
100 g (3½ oz) mango
100 g (3½ oz) banana

Juice the pineapple, grapes, orange and apple. Whizz in a blender with
the mango, banana and a couple of ice cubes for a super sweet smoothie.
Serve decorated with orange wedges and mint.

makes 400 ml (14 fl oz)

good for
weight gain

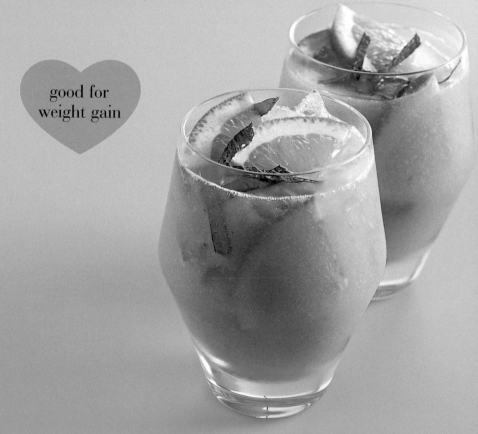

pear, prune & spinach

250 g (8 oz) pear
25 g (1 oz) pitted prunes
125 g (4 oz) spinach

Juice all the ingredients and serve in a glass over ice cubes. Decorate with pear slices, if liked.

makes 200 ml (7 fl oz)

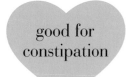

good for
constipation

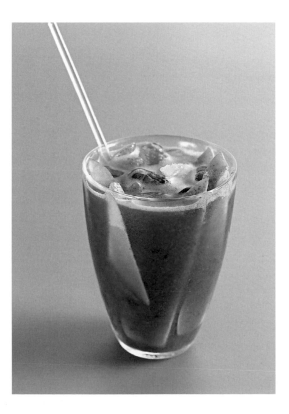

ginger spice

300 g (10 oz) carrot
50 g (2 oz) fennel
75 g (3 oz) celery
2.5 cm (1 inch) cube fresh root
    ginger, roughly chopped
1 tablespoon spirulina (optional)

Juice the ingredients and serve
over ice. If liked, decorate with
strips of fennel and fennel fronds.
Good to kickstart a diet.

makes 200 ml (7 fl oz)

apple & blueberry

250 g (8 oz) apple
125 g (4 oz) blueberries, fresh
    or frozen

Juice the apple, then whizz in a
blender with the blueberries.
Serve in a tumbler.

makes 150 ml (5 fl oz)

ginger zinger

125 g (4 oz) carrot
250 g (8 oz) cantaloupe melon
1 lime
2.5 cm (1 inch) cube fresh root
    ginger, roughly chopped

Juice the carrot, melon, lime and
ginger. Serve in a glass over ice.
Decorate with lime wedges and
seeds from a cardamom pod, if
liked.

makes 200 ml (7 fl oz)

orange & banana smoothie

150 g (5 oz) carrot
100 g (3½ oz) orange
100 g (3½ oz) banana
1 dried apricot

Juice the carrot and orange. Whizz
in a blender with the banana,
apricot and some ice cubes.
Decorate with chunks of banana,
if liked. Wards off colds.

makes 200 ml (7 fl oz)

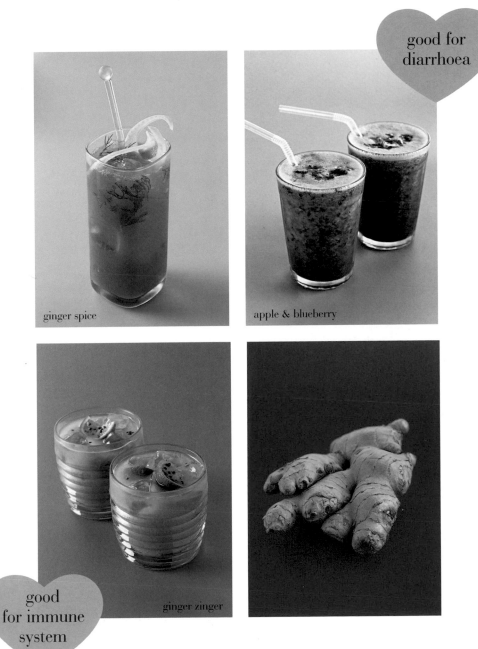

ginger spice

apple & blueberry

good for
diarrhoea

ginger zinger

good
for immune
system

sweet & sour

1 mango
1 orange
125 g (4 oz) cranberries
100 ml (3½ fl oz) water
1 teaspoon clear honey

Juice all the fruit, pour the juice into a glass and stir in the water and honey. Add a couple of ice cubes if desired and drink immediately.

makes 200 ml (7 fl oz)

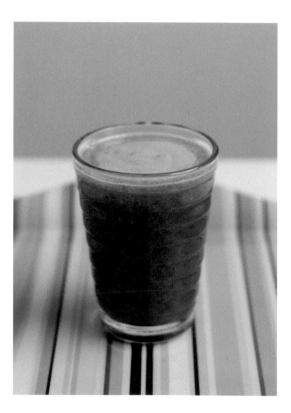

fends off
colds

carrot, chicory & celery

175 g (6 oz) carrot
125 g (4 oz) chicory
125 g (4 oz) celery

Juice the carrot, chicory and celery. Whizz in a blender with a couple of ice cubes and serve decorated with lemon slices and some chopped parsley, if liked.

makes 200 ml (7 fl oz)

good for
eyesight

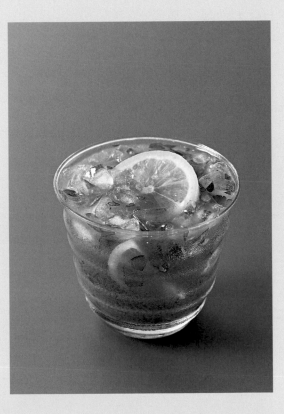

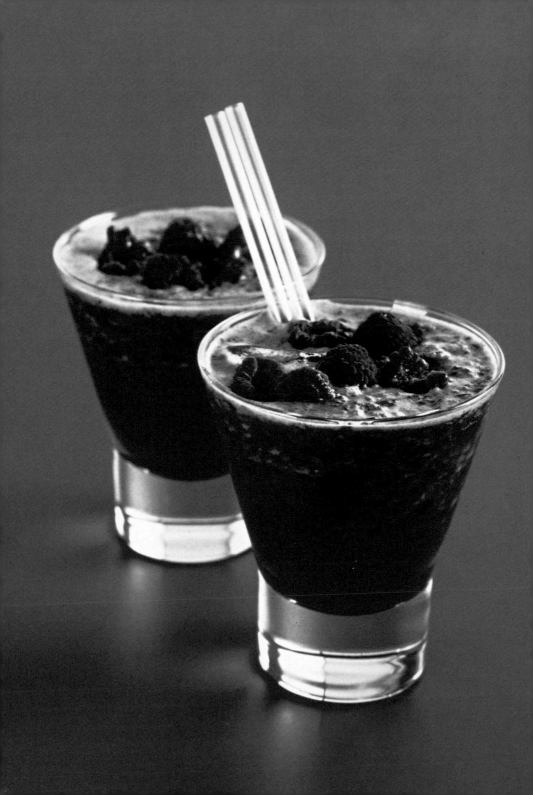

grapefruit, kiwifruit & berry

150 g (5 oz) grapefruit
50 g (2 oz) kiwifruit
175 g (6 oz) pineapple
50 g (2 oz) frozen raspberries
50 g (2 oz) frozen cranberries

Juice the grapefruit, kiwifruit and pineapple. Whizz in a blender with the frozen berries. Decorate with raspberries, if liked, and serve with straws.

makes 200 ml (7 fl oz)

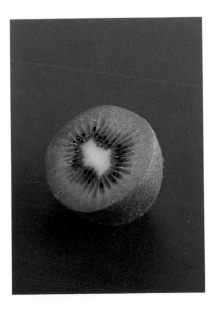

parsnip, pepper & cucumber (left)

175 g (6 oz) parsnip
175 g (6 oz) green pepper
100 g (3½ oz) watercress
175 g (6 oz) cucumber

Juice the ingredients together and serve over ice with a sprinkling of mint.

makes 200 ml (7 fl oz)

potato, radish & carrot (right)

100 g (3½ oz) potato
100 g (3½ oz) radish
100 g (3½ oz) carrot
100 g (3½ oz) cucumber

Juice the ingredients together and whizz in a blender with two ice cubes.
Serve in a tall glass decorated with radish slices, if liked.

makes 200 ml (7 fl oz)

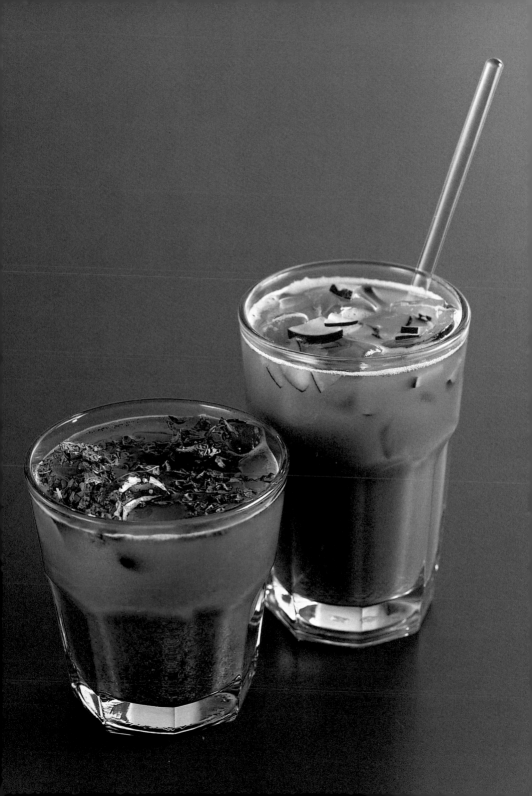

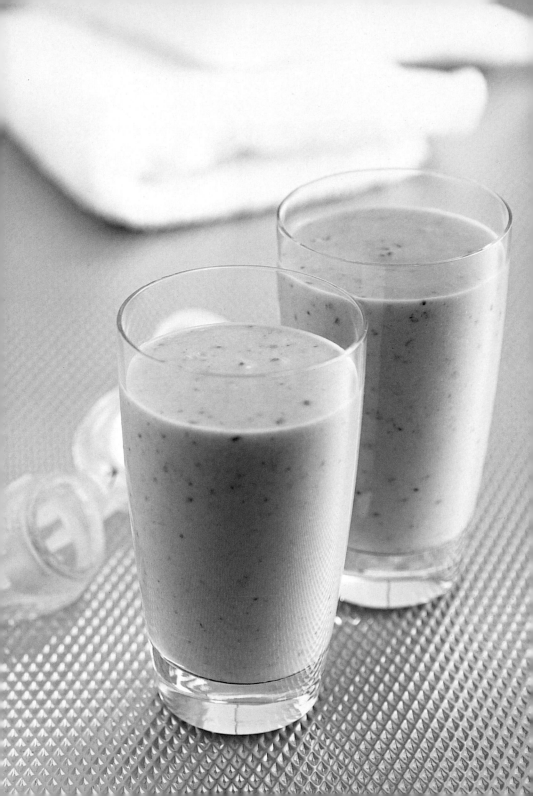

dried fruit salad smoothie

125 g (4 oz) dried fruit salad
400 ml (15 fl oz) apple juice, more if necessary
200 ml (7 fl oz) Greek yogurt

Roughly chop the fruit and place in a large bowl. Pour over the apple juice, cover and allow to stand overnight. Put the mixture in a blender, add the yogurt and process until smooth, adding a little more apple juice if necessary. Serve immediately.

makes 400 ml (14 fl oz)

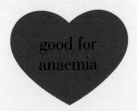

good for
anaemia

stress buster

150 g (5 oz) spinach
150 g (5 oz) broccoli
2 tomatoes

Juice the spinach, broccoli and
tomatoes then mix together. Serve
in a tumbler over ice, decorated
with sliced tomatoes, if liked.

makes 200 ml (7 fl oz)

grapefruit, carrot & spinach

125 g (4 oz) pink grapefruit
125 g (4 oz) carrot
125 g (4 oz) spinach

Peel the grapefruit, keeping as
much of the pith as possible. Juice
all the ingredients and serve with
slices of grapefruit, if liked.

makes 200 ml (7 fl oz)

pineapple & parsnip shake

250 g (8 oz) pineapple
100 g (3½ oz) parsnip
100 g (3½ oz) carrot
75 ml (3 fl oz) soya milk

Juice the pineapple, parsnip and
carrot. Whizz in a blender with
the soya milk and a couple of ice
cubes. Decorate with pineapple
wedges, if liked. Aids digestion.

makes 200 ml (7 fl oz)

pepper, tomato & parsley

175 g (6 oz) red pepper
175 g (6 oz) tomatoes
100 g (3½ oz) white cabbage
1 tablespoon chopped parsley

Juice the pepper, tomatoes and
cabbage. Pour into a tall glass, stir
in the parsley and decorate with a
lime wedge, if liked.

makes 200 ml (7 fl oz)

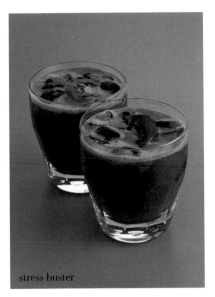

stress buster

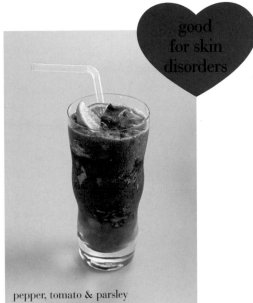

pepper, tomato & parsley

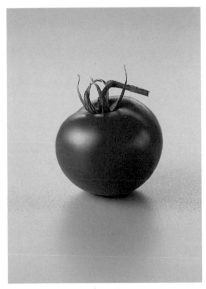

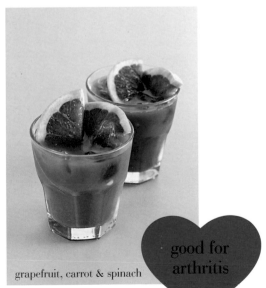

grapefruit, carrot & spinach

lettuce, root veg & melon

125 g (4 oz) carrot
125 g (4 oz) lettuce
125 g (4 oz) parsnip
125 g (4 oz) cantaloupe melon

Juice the carrot, lettuce and parsnip with the flesh of the melon. Serve in a tall glass with wedges of melon, if liked.

makes 200 ml (7 fl oz)

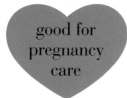

good for
pregnancy
care

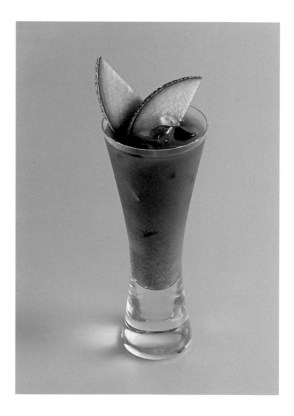

watermelon & strawberry

200 g (7 oz) watermelon
200 g (7 oz) strawberries

Juice the fruit and whizz in a blender with a couple of ice cubes. Serve decorated with mint leaves and whole or sliced strawberries, if liked.

makes 200 ml (7 fl oz)

good for
detoxifying

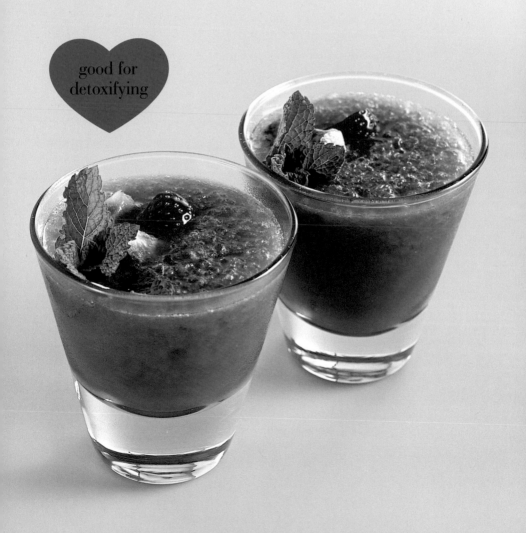

energy

Natural juices and smoothies are great for sports people because they delivery fluid, energy-giving carbohydrate and a wealth of other important nutrients all in one glass. They will give a beneficial boost before, during and especially after exercise, a time when sports people can lose their appetite for solid food. So, whether you are a marathon runner or play a weekly game of tennis, these recipes will help you get more from your exercise routine.

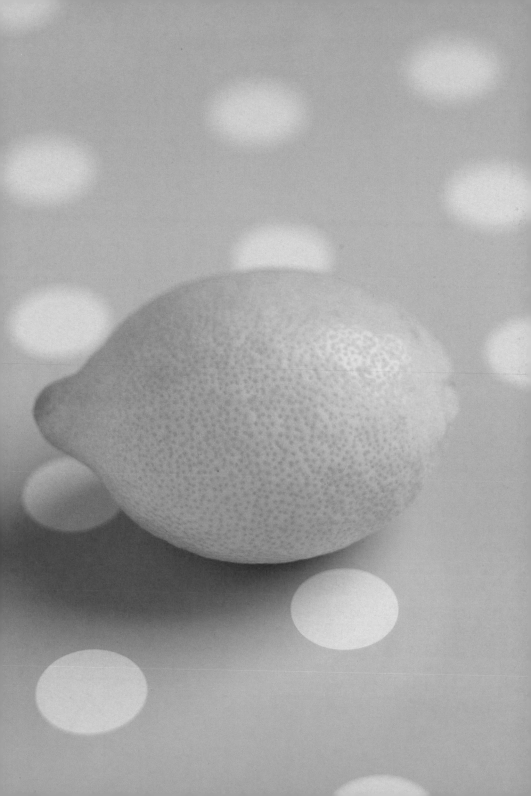

celery, apple & alfalfa

3 celery sticks
2 tart-flavoured apples, such as Granny Smith
1 cup alfalfa

Feed all the ingredients into a juicer in alternating batches. Pour into a glass, add a couple of ice cubes, and drink immediately.

makes 250 ml (8 fl oz)

perfect for
pre-exercise

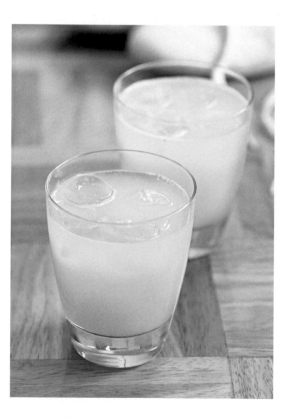

banana & almond smoothie

2 very ripe bananas
450 ml (¾ pint) soya milk
40 g (1½ oz) ground almonds
pinch of ground cinnamon
a little honey (optional)

Slice the bananas and freeze for at least 2 hours or overnight. Place the frozen bananas, soya milk, ground almonds and cinnamon in a blender, add the honey, if using, and process until thick and frothy. Pour into glasses, add a couple of ice cubes and decorate with ground cinnamon, if liked.

makes 600 ml (1 pint)

good for
endurance
sport

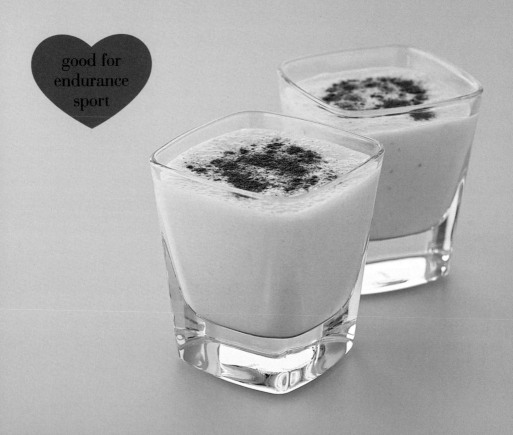

mango, melon & orange

1 ripe mango
½ galia melon
200 ml (7 fl oz) orange juice

Place the mango and melon flesh in a blender. Add the orange juice and a couple of ice cubes, then purée until smooth. Serve immediately.

makes 400 ml (14 fl oz)

good for
busy kids on
the go

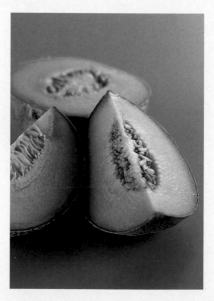

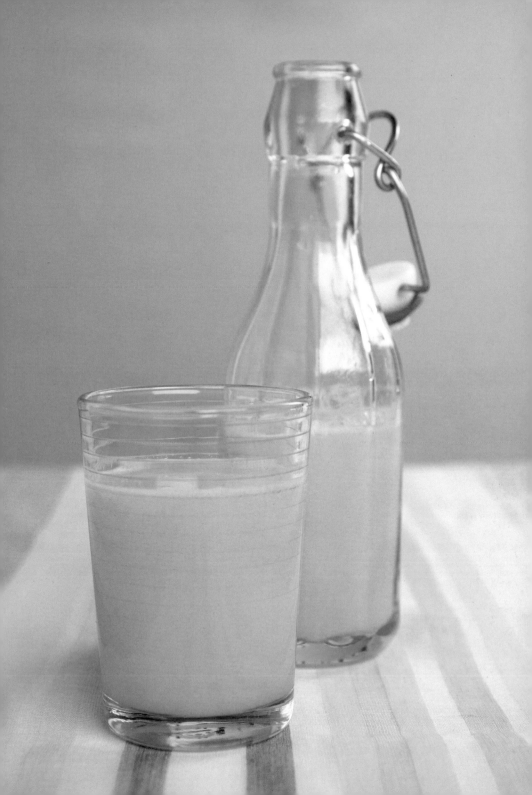

kiwifruit, melon & passion fruit smoothie

¼ watermelon, about 300 g (10 oz) flesh
2 kiwifruit
175 ml (6 fl oz) passion fruit juice

Remove and discard the seeds from the watermelon and dice the flesh.
Put it in a freezer container and freeze for at least 2 hours or overnight.
Peel and roughly chop the kiwifruit and place in a blender with the
watermelon and the passion fruit juice and process until thick. Serve
immediately.

makes 400 ml (14 fl oz)

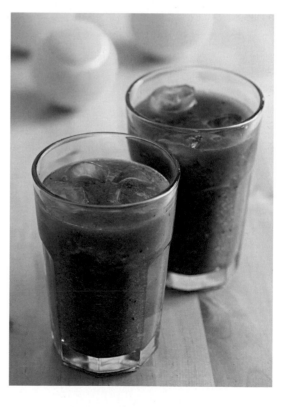

beneficial
after most
exercise

the rehydrator

1 orange
50 g (2 oz) cucumber
100 ml (3½ fl oz) cranberry juice

Juice the orange (with as much of its pith as possible) and cucumber. Mix this juice with the cranberry juice. Serve in a tall glass over ice, decorated with slices of cucumber, if liked.

makes 200 ml (7 fl oz)

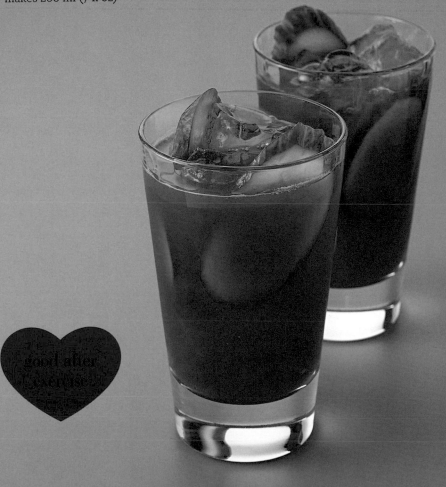

good after exercise

sweet potato, orange & carrot

1 small sweet potato
2 small oranges
1 large carrot

Juice the sweet potato, oranges and carrots. To make a smoother, creamier drink, transfer the juice to a blender and process with a couple of ice cubes. Decorate with mint sprigs, if liked.

makes 200 ml (7 fl oz)

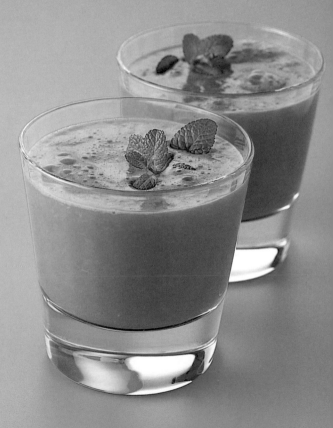

banana & peanut butter smoothie

1 ripe banana
300 ml (10 fl oz) semi-skimmed milk
1 tablespoon smooth peanut butter
   or 2 teaspoons tahini paste

Peel and slice the banana, put it in a freezer container and freeze for at
least 2 hours or overnight. Put the banana, milk and peanut butter or tahini
paste in a food processor or blender and process until smooth. Serve
immediately.

makes 400 ml (14 fl oz)

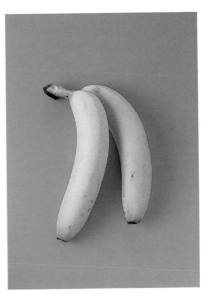

great
boost after
exercise

watermelon, lime & orange

¼ watermelon, about 300 g (10 oz) flesh
2 oranges
zest and juice of ½ lime

Juice the fruit, stir in the lime zest and juice, pour it into a glass, and add a couple of ice cubes. Decorate with slices of orange, if desired.

makes 300 ml (10 fl oz)

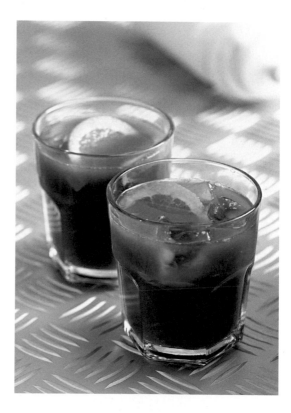

has vitamin
C for muscle
function

melon, pineapple & apple

½ galia melon
¼ pineapple, about 215 g (7½ oz)
1 green apple

Juice the flesh of the melon and pineapple with the apple. Pour into a glass and add a couple of ice cubes. Decorate with apple slices, if liked.

makes 300 ml (10 fl oz)

high carb
content for
fuel

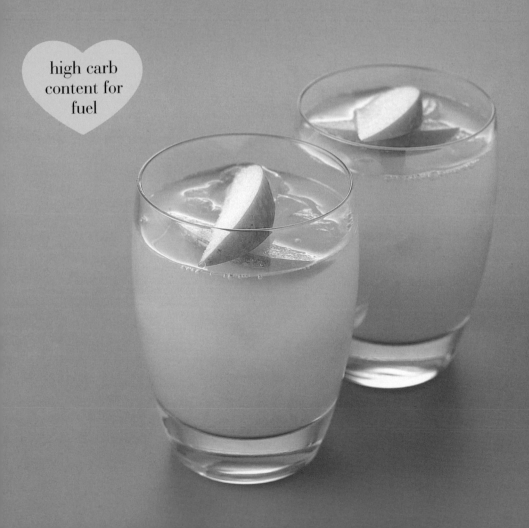

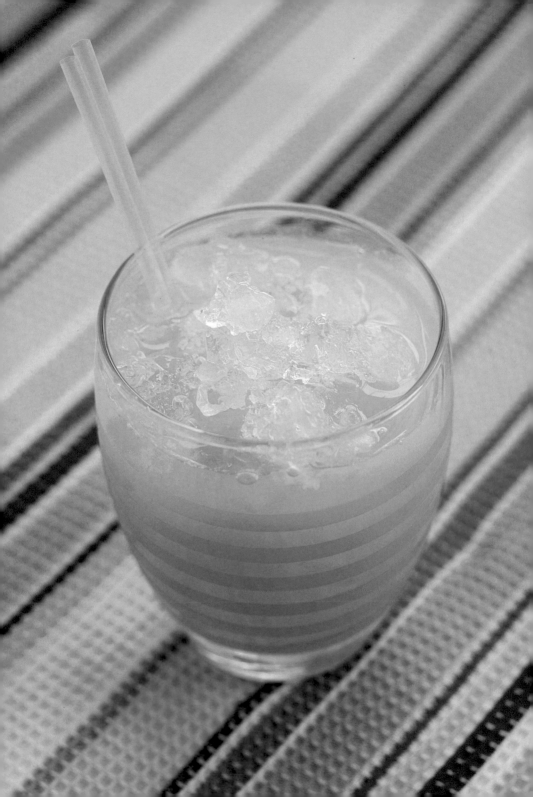

mango cooler

100 g (3½ oz) mango
200 g (7 oz) apple, peeled
125 g (4 oz) cucumber, peeled

Juice the ingredients and blend together with a couple of ice cubes.

makes 200 ml (7 fl oz)

cooling drink
for active
kids

carrot, apple & ginger

2 carrots
1 tart-flavoured apple, such as Granny Smith
½ inch cube fresh root ginger, roughly chopped

Juice all the ingredients, pour into a glass and add a couple of ice cubes.

makes 250 ml (8 fl oz)

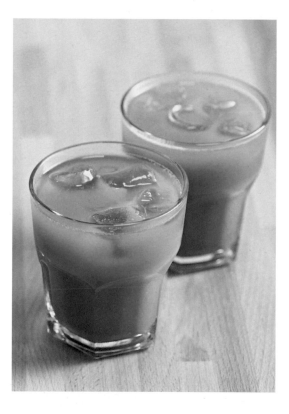

ideal during
yoga or when
walking

apple, mango & passion fruit

3 apples, preferably red
1 mango
2 passion fruit

Juice the apples and mango with the passion fruit flesh (discard the
seeds). Pour the juice into a glass and add a couple of ice cubes. Decorate
with apple slices, if liked.

makes 300 ml (10 fl oz)

good before
an endurance
event

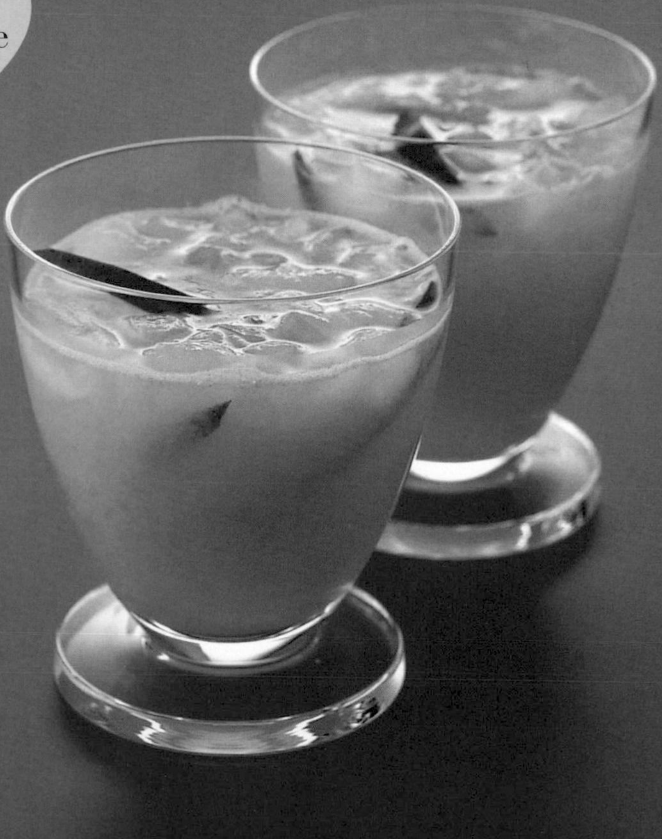

pear & apple chiller

2 pears
1 apple
40 g (1½ oz) watercress

Choose ripe pears if possible. Feed the pear and apple chunks and the watercress into the juicer in alternate batches. Pour into a glass and add ice cubes. Decorate with watercress leaves, if liked.

makes 250 ml (8 fl oz)

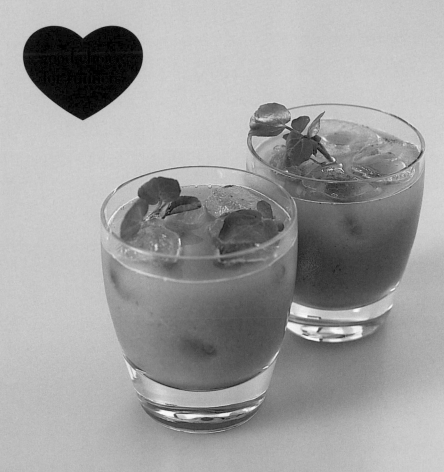

strawberry, kiwi & banana

250 g (8 oz) strawberries
1 kiwifruit
½ large banana
1 tablespoon spirulina
1 tablespoon linseeds

Juice the strawberries and kiwifruit and whizz in a blender with the banana, spirulina, linseeds and a couple of ice cubes. Decorate with redcurrants and linseeds, if liked.

makes 200 ml (7 fl oz)

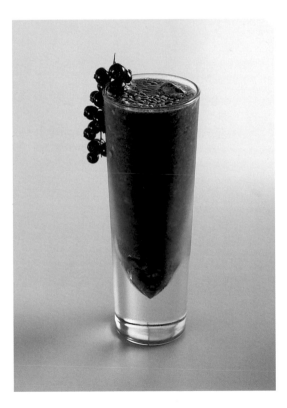

carrot & kiwifruit

2 carrots
1 kiwifruit

Juice the carrots and kiwifruit. Pour into a glass and add a couple of ice cubes. Decorate with slices of kiwifruit, if desired.

makes 250 ml (8 fl oz)

orange & raspberry

2 large oranges
175 g (6 oz) raspberries
250 ml (8 fl oz) water

Juice the fruit then add the water. Pour into a glass and add a couple of ice cubes.

makes 500 ml (17 fl oz)

beetroot, apple & carrot

2 small beetroot, about 100 g (3½ oz)
1 carrot
2 apples
300 ml (10 fl oz) water

Juice the beetroot, carrot and apples. Add the water, mix well then pour into a glass. Add a couple of ice cubes to chill.

makes 600 ml (1 pint)

spinach, carrot & tomato

large handful of baby spinach
2 carrots
4 tomatoes
½ red pepper

Juice the vegetables in alternating batches. Serve with ice.

makes 300 ml (10 fl oz)

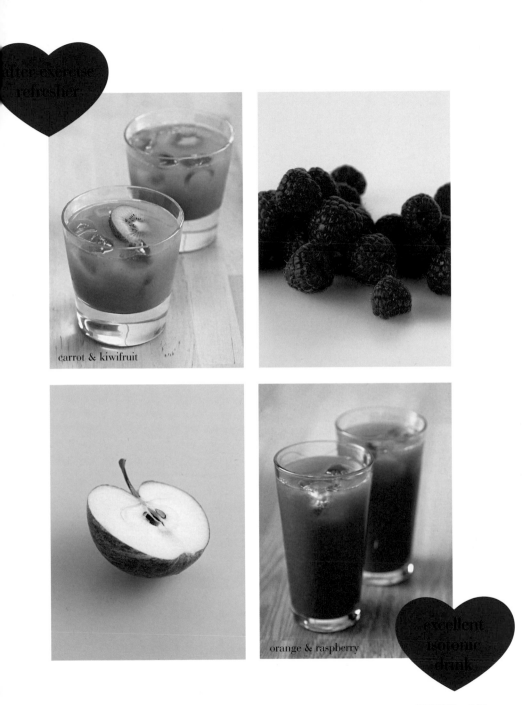

after exercise refresher

carrot & kiwifruit

orange & raspberry

excellent isotonic drink

energy 151

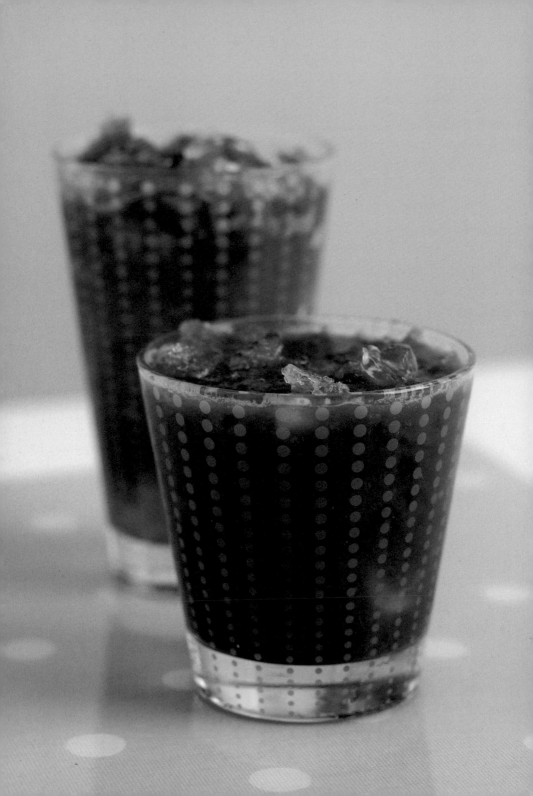

watermelon & raspberry

300 g (10 oz) watermelon
125 g (4 oz) raspberries

Juice all the fruit, pour into a glass and add some crushed ice
cubes if desired.

makes 200 ml (7 fl oz)

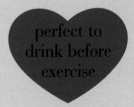

perfect to
drink before
exercise

spicy celery, tomato & red pepper

3 tomatoes, about 500 g (1 lb)
4 celery sticks
½ red pepper
½ red chilli (optional)
1 garlic clove, crushed (optional)

Choose ripe tomatoes if possible. Juice them with the celery and red pepper. Pour into a glass, stir in the chilli and crushed garlic, if using, and add a couple of ice cubes, if liked.

makes 300 ml (10 fl oz)

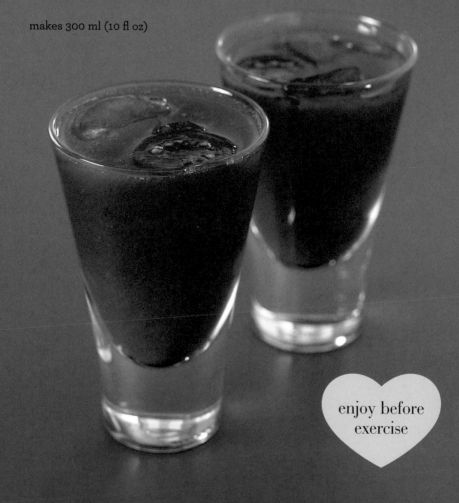

enjoy before exercise

pink grapefruit & pineapple

1 pink grapefruit
¼ pineapple, about 215 g (7½ oz)
350 ml (12 fl oz) water

Juice the fruit then add the water. Pour into a glass and add a couple of ice cubes.

makes 600 ml (1 pint)

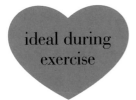

ideal during exercise

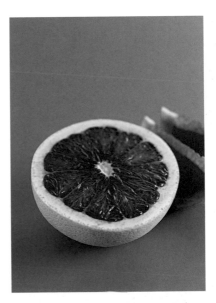

pear, kiwifruit & lime

2 ripe pears
3 kiwifruit
½ lime

Juice all the ingredients. Pour into a glass, add a couple of ice cubes, and decorate with slices of pear, if desired.

makes 300 ml (10 fl oz)

protects
against muscle
damage

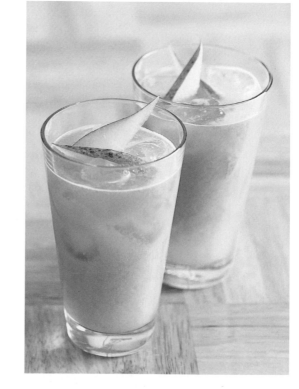

melon & grape

½ galia melon
175 g (6 oz) green grapes
300 ml (10 fl oz) water

Juice the melon flesh with the grapes. Mix in the water and pour into two
glasses. Add a couple of ice cubes and decorate with grapes, if liked.

makes 600 ml (1 pint)

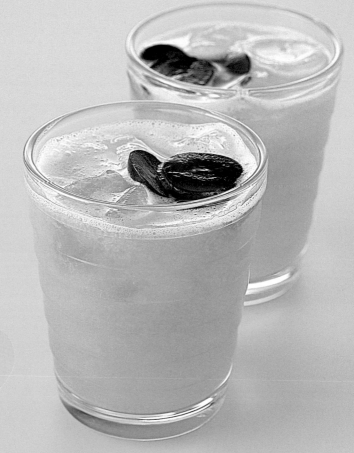

good during
endurance
activities

kiwifruit & grape

2 kiwifruit, peeled
300 g (10 oz) green grapes

Juice the kiwifruit flesh with the grapes. Pour the juice into a glass and add some crushed ice. Decorate with kiwifruit, if liked.

makes 300 ml (10 fl oz)

with vitamin
C to protect
muscles

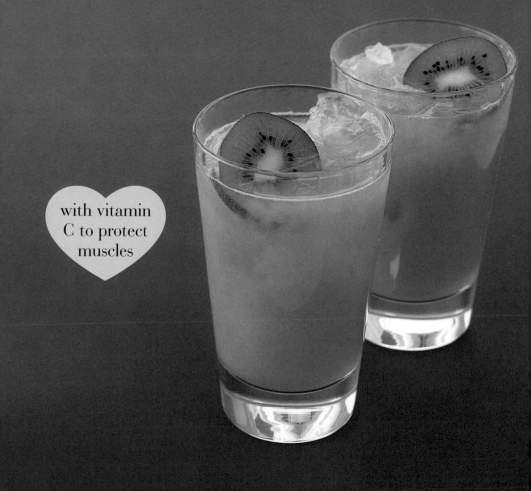

strawberry & kiwifruit

150 g (5 oz) strawberries
2 kiwifruit

Wash and hull the strawberries. Peel the kiwifruit and slice them into even-size pieces. Juice the fruit, pour it into a glass then add a couple of ice cubes, if desired.

makes 300 ml (10 fl oz)

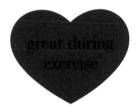

great during
exercise

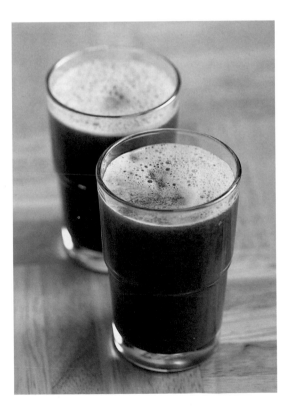

mango, pineapple & lime smoothie

1 ripe mango
300 ml (10 fl oz) pineapple juice
zest and juice of ½ lime

Peel the mango, remove the pit, roughly chop the flesh and put it in a freezer container. Freeze for at least 2 hours or overnight. Place the frozen mango in a food processor or blender with the pineapple juice and lime zest and juice and process until thick. Decorate with lime wedges, if desired, and serve immediately.

makes 400 ml (14 fl oz)

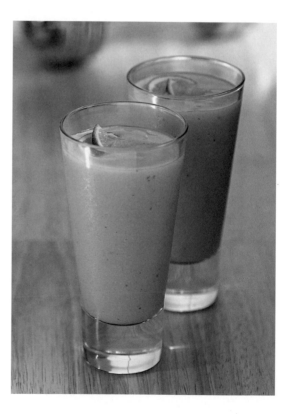

good after
exercise

energy burst

125 g (4 oz) spinach
250 g (8 oz) apple
100 g (3½ oz) yellow pepper
a pinch of cinnamon

Juice all the ingredients and serve in a glass. If liked, add a cinnamon stick for decoration.

makes 200 ml (7 fl oz)

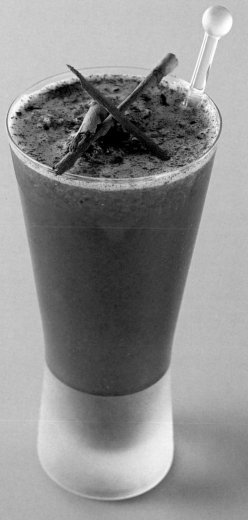

strawberry & cherry sparkler

150 g (5 oz) strawberries
125 g (4 oz) cherries
125 g (4 oz) watermelon
100 ml (3½ fl oz) orange juice
500 ml (17 fl oz) sparkling water, chilled

Deseed the watermelon and cut it into small chunks. Put all the fruit in a blender with the orange juice and blend until smooth. If you don't like 'bits' in your drink, sieve the fruit purée over a bowl to remove the pips, skin and seeds. Pour the purée into the glasses. Top up with the sparkling water.

makes 600 ml (1 pint)

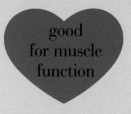

good
for muscle
function

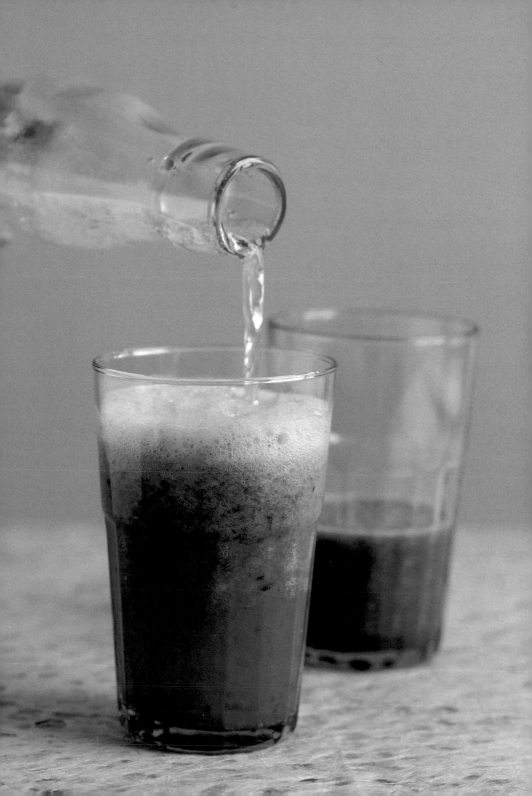

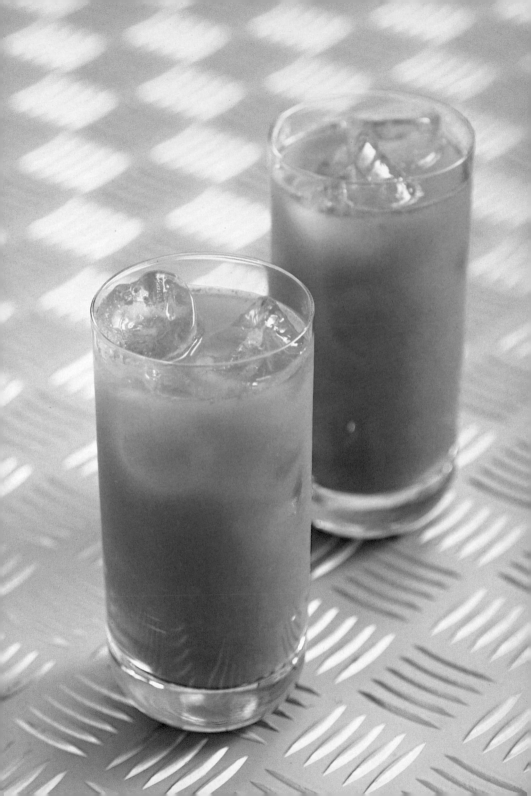

carrot, orange & apple

2 carrots
1 orange
1 tart-flavored apple, such as Granny Smith

Cut the carrots and apple into even-size pieces. Juice all the fruit, pour into a glass, then add a couple of ice cubes.

makes 250 ml (8 fl oz)

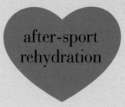

after-sport
rehydration

strawberry refresher

215 g (7½ oz) strawberries
150 g (5 oz) redcurrants
1 orange
250 ml (8 fl oz) water
1 teaspoon clear honey (optional)
½ tablespoon wheatgerm (optional)

Peel the orange and divide it into segments. Juice the fruit, then add the water. Pour into a glass, stir in the honey and wheatgerm, if using, and add a couple of ice cubes, if desired.

makes 475 ml (17 fl oz)

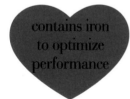

contains iron
to optimize
performance

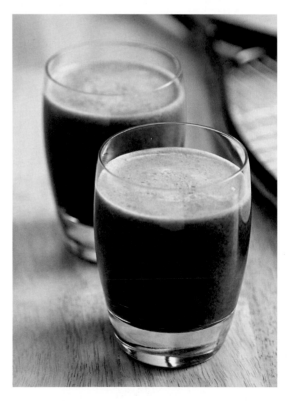

apple & plum

5 ripe plums
3 red apples

Cut the apples into even-size pieces. Juice the fruit and serve in a glass over a couple of ice cubes.

makes 300 ml (10 fl oz)

strawberry, peach & apple

125 g (4 oz) strawberries
2 peaches
1 red apple
300 ml (10 fl oz) water

Juice all the fruit. Add the water, then pour the juice into a glass and add a couple of ice cubes, if desired.

makes 600 ml (1 pint)

cucumber & mint lassi

200 g (7 oz) cucumber
250 ml (8 fl oz) natural bio yogurt
handful of chopped mint
¼ teaspoon salt (optional)

Slice the cucumber in half lengthwise and, using a teaspoon, remove and discard the seeds. Roughly chop the flesh and place it in a food processor or blender with the yogurt, mint, and salt, if using, and process until smooth. Pour into a glass, add a couple of ice cubes, decorate with mint, if desired, and drink immediately.

makes 300 ml (10 fl oz)

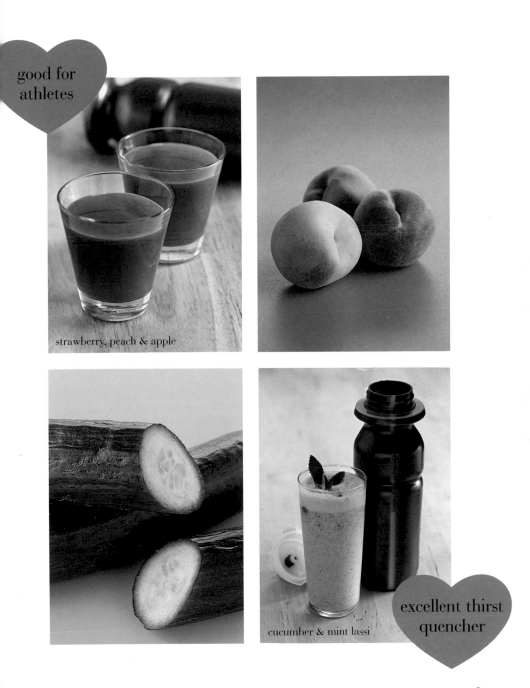

good for athletes

strawberry, peach & apple

cucumber & mint lassi

excellent thirst quencher

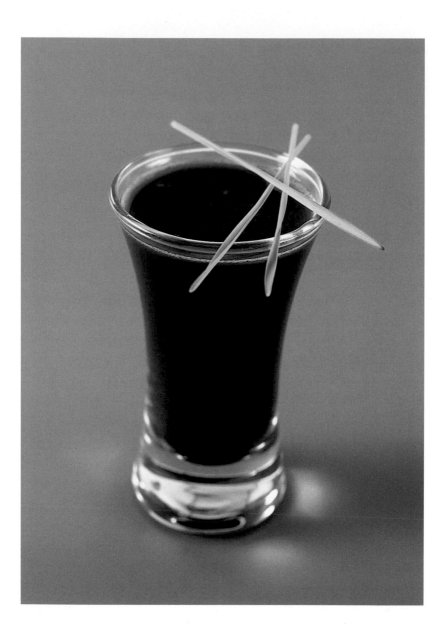

kale, wheatgrass & spirulina

25 g (1 oz) kale
100 g (3½ oz) wheatgrass
1 teaspoon spirulina

Juice the kale and the wheatgrass then stir in the spirulina powder.
Serve in a small glass decorated with wheatgrass blades.

makes 50 ml (2 fl oz)

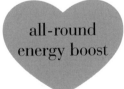

all-round
energy boost

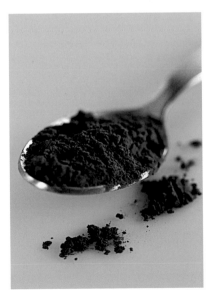

banana, strawberry & pineapple smoothie

1 small ripe banana
75 g (3 oz) strawberries
250 ml (8 fl oz) pineapple juice

Peel and slice the banana. Wash, hull and roughly chop the strawberries. Place the fruit into a freezer container and freeze for at least 2 hours or overnight. Place the frozen fruit and the pineapple juice in a food processor or blender and process until thick. Decorate with strawberries, if desired, and serve immediately.

makes 400 ml (14 fl oz)

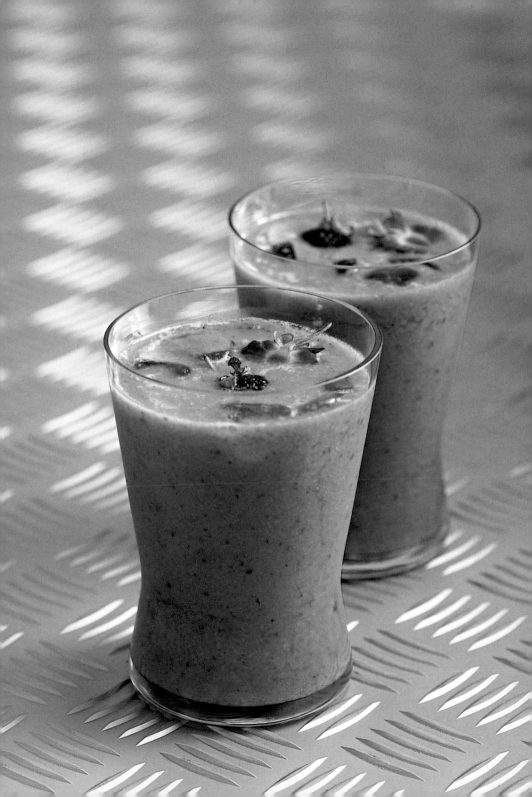

blackberry & grape smoothie

125 g (4 oz) frozen raspberries
300 ml (10 fl oz) purple grape juice
3 tablespoons Quark or fromage frais
1 teaspoon clear honey (optional)

Put the blackberries, grape juice, and Quark or fromage frais in a food processor or blender, add the honey, if using, and process until thick. Decorate with a few blackberries and serve immediately.

makes 400 ml (14 fl oz)

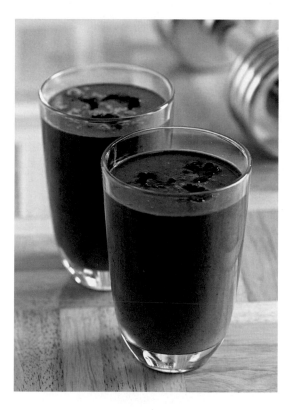

melon, kiwifruit & grape

½ honeydew melon
2 kiwifruit, peeled
125 g (4 oz) green grapes

Juice the flesh of the melon and kiwifruit with the grapes. Pour into a glass
and add ice cubes. Serve with slices of kiwifruit, if liked.

makes 300 ml (10 fl oz)

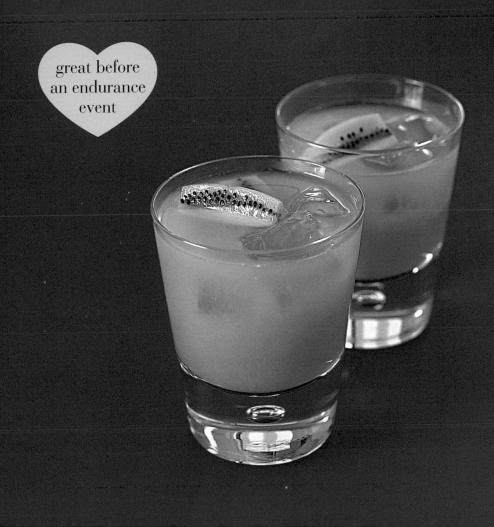

great before
an endurance
event

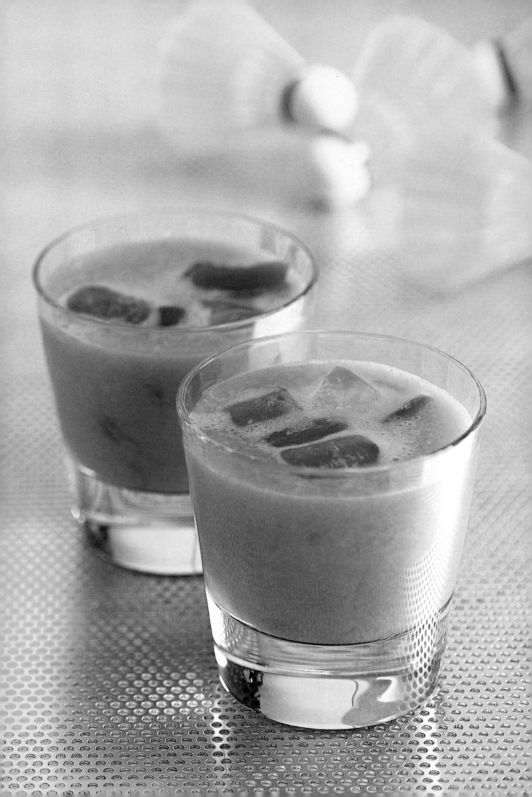

apricot & pineapple smoothie

65 g (2½ oz) ready-to-eat apricots
350 ml (12 fl oz) pineapple juice

Roughly chop the apricots into small pieces and put them in a large
bowl. Pour the pineapple juice over them, cover the bowl, and allow to
stand overnight. Tip the contents of the bowl into a food processor or
blender and process until smooth. Add a couple of ice cubes and drink
immediately.

makes 350 ml (12 fl oz)

boosts
depleted energy
levels

avocado & banana smoothie

1 small ripe avocado
1 small ripe banana
250 ml (8 fl oz) skimmed milk

Place the avocado flesh, banana and milk in a food processor or blender and process until smooth. Pour into a glass, add a couple of ice cubes and drink immediately.

makes 400 ml (14 fl oz)

orange, apple & pear

2 oranges
1 red apple
1 pear
1 teaspoon clear honey (optional)

Juice the fruit and pour it into a glass. Stir in the honey, if using, and add a couple of ice cubes.

makes 350 ml (11 fl oz)

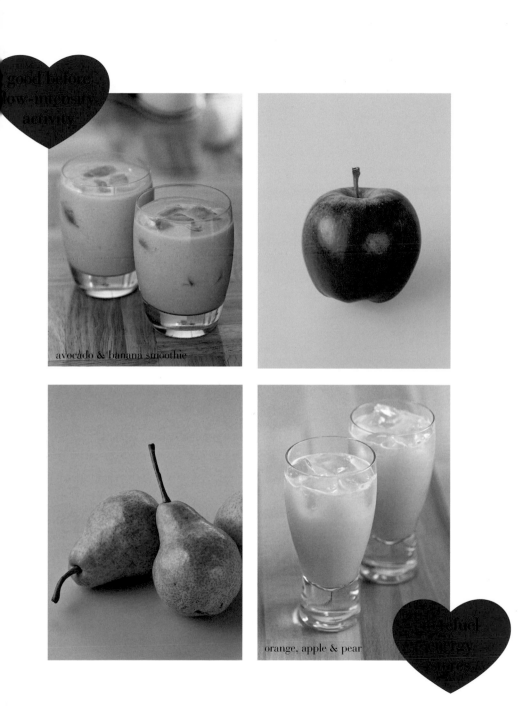

good before low-intensity activity

avocado & banana smoothie

orange, apple & pear

the fuel that energy stores

tropical fruit smoothie

1 large banana
1 large ripe mango
160 ml (5 fl oz) natural bio yogurt
300 ml (10 fl oz) pineapple juice

Peel and slice the banana, then put it in a freezer container and freeze for at least 2 hours or overnight. Peel the mango, remove the pit and roughly chop the flesh. Place it in a food processor or blender with the frozen banana, yogurt, and pineapple juice. Process until smooth and serve immediately, decorated with pineapple cubes, if desired.

makes 600 ml (1 pint)

good source
of carbs for
fuel

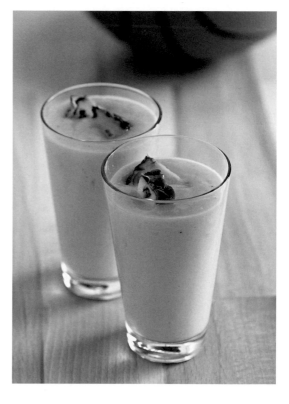

power pack

3 small carrots
2 beetroot, about 125 g (4 oz)
1 orange
125 g (4 oz) strawberries

Juice the carrots, beetroots and orange together. Put the juice into a blender with a couple of ice cubes and the strawberries. Whizz for 20 seconds and serve in a tall glass. Decorate with strips of orange rind, if liked.

makes 200 ml (7 fl oz)

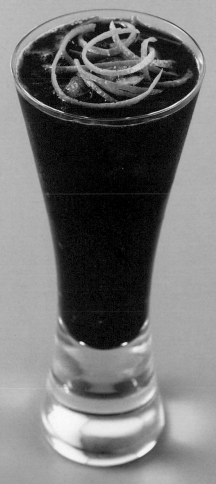

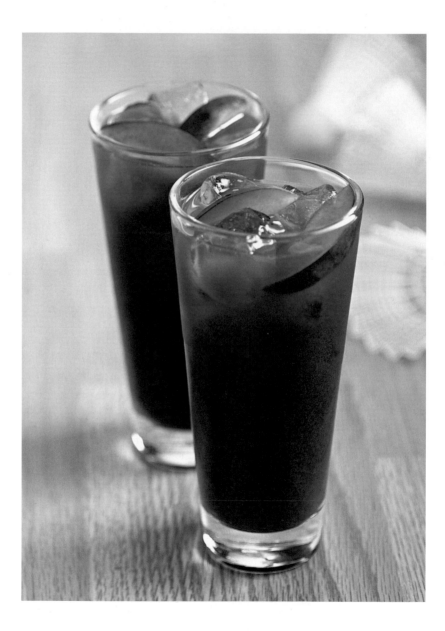

grape & plum

150 g (5 oz) red grapes
5 plums, about 10 oz

Juice the fruit, pour it into a glass, and add a couple of ice cubes. Decorate with slices of plum, if desired.

makes 300 ml (10 fl oz)

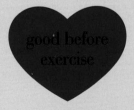

good before
exercise

banana & mango smoothie

1 ripe banana
1 ripe mango
175 ml (6 fl oz) orange juice
175 ml (6 fl oz) semi-skimmed milk
3 tablespoons natural yogurt

Peel and slice the banana, then put it in a freezer container and freeze for at least 2 hours or overnight. Place the mango flesh in a food processor or blender with the frozen banana, yogurt and pineapple juice. Process until smooth and serve immediately, decorated with pineapple cubes, if desired.

makes 475 ml (17 fl oz)

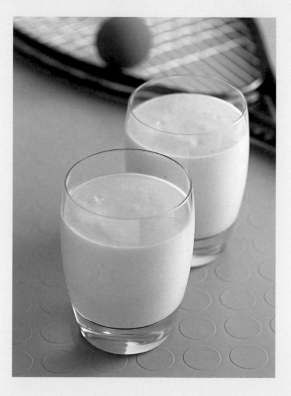

good for nerve
and muscle
function

apricot & orange smoothie

13 oz can apricots in natural juice, drained
160 ml (5 fl oz) apricot or natural yogurt
175 ml (6 fl oz) orange juice

Place the apricots in a food processor or blender with the yogurt and
orange juice and process until smooth. Pour into a glass over a couple of
ice cubes and serve sprinkled with a little cinnamon, if desired.

makes 475 ml (17 fl oz)

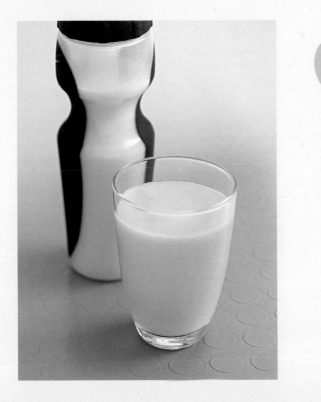

good for fluid
replacement

orange, mango & strawberry smoothie

25 g (4 oz) strawberries
1 small ripe mango
300 ml (10 fl oz) orange juice

Hull the strawberries, place them in a freezer container and freeze for
2 hours or overnight. Place the mango flesh in a food processor or blender
with the strawberries and orange juice and process until thick. Decorate
with slices of orange, if desired, and serve immediately.

makes 400 ml (14 fl oz)

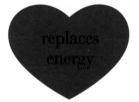

replaces
energy

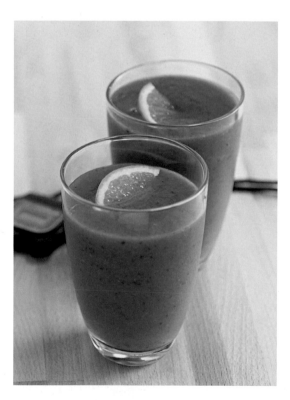

red velvet

½ large red pepper, deseeded
125 g (4 oz) strawberries
½ small tomato, about 50 g (2 oz)
½ large mango
⅛ watermelon, about 125 g (4 oz) flesh

Juice all the ingredients, then whizz in a blender with 3 ice cubes and
serve in a tall glass. Decorate with mango slices, if liked.

makes 200 ml (7 fl oz)

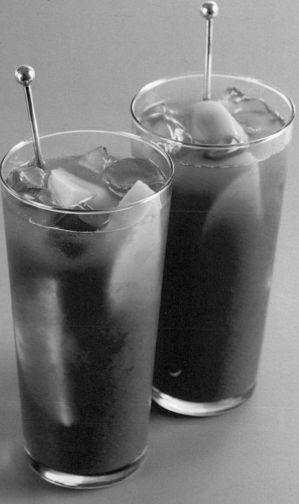

index

conversion chart

weights

5g	¼oz
15g	½oz
20g	¾oz
25g	1oz
50g	2oz
65g	2½oz
75g	3oz
125g	4oz
150g	5oz
175g	6oz
200g	7oz
250g	8oz
275g	9oz
300g	10oz
325g	11oz
375g	12oz
400g	13oz
425g	14oz
450g	14½oz
475g	15oz
500g	1lb
625g	1¼lb
750g	1½lb
875g	1¾lb
1kg	2lb

teaspoons

1 tsp	5g
1 tbsp	15g
1 tsp	5ml
1 tbsp	15ml

liquids

15ml	½fl oz
25ml	1fl oz
50ml	2fl oz
75ml	3fl oz
10ml	3½fl oz
125ml	4fl oz
150ml	¼ pint
175ml	6fl oz
200ml	7fl oz
250ml	8fl oz
275ml	9fl oz
300ml	½ pint
325ml	11fl oz
350ml	12fl oz
375ml	13fl oz
400ml	14fl oz
450ml	¾ pint
475ml	16fl oz
500ml	17fl oz
575ml	18fl oz
600ml	1 pint
750ml	1¼ pints
900ml	1½ pints
1 litre	1¾ pints